CHANGE YOUR MIND

About the Author

RJ Spina is a true leader and metaphysical teacher, and the world has never needed one so desperately. He has verifiably healed himself of permanent chest-down paralysis, severe chronic illness, and life-threatening conditions through his own authentic transcendence. His teachings, wisdom, guidance, and revolutionary self-healing and self-realization techniques have already completely changed and saved the lives of many across the globe. He has dedicated his life to the freeing and healing of humanity on all levels.

As a child, RJ would naturally access the limitless, hidden realms beyond our ordinary sensory perception. He always felt a deep sense of knowingness that went well beyond the human intellect. Upon turning twenty-four and struggling with "normal" life, he found himself in an unforced and naturally deep state of meditation. That moment was a turning point in this life as RJ. What he tangibly experienced and authentically understood was the beginning of his own liberation and self-realization.

RJ currently lives in Canandaigua, NY, with his partner and their Jack Russell/Chihuahua, Sophia. He is the founder and president of the nonprofit Human Advancement through Higher Consciousness and the author of the best-selling book *Supercharged Self-Healing* and the upcoming book *Change Your Mind* (August 2023, Llewellyn Worldwide and Blackstone Audible Publishing). He teaches revolutionary self-healing, self-realization, and the real magick of manifestation and counsels people worldwide.

Website: https://www.ascendthefrequencies.com/
Instagram: https://www.instagram.com/ascendthefrequencies12/
Facebook: https://www.facebook.com/ascendthefrequencies12/
YouTube: https://www.youtube.com/@rjspinaascendthefrequencie4584

Other Books by RJ Spina

Supercharged Self-Healing

FIRST EDITION
Fourth Printing, 2024

Cover design by Shannon McKuhen

Llewellyn Publications is a registered trademark of Llewellyn Worldwide Ltd.

Library of Congress Cataloging-in-Publication Data
Names: Spina, RJ, author.
Title: Change your mind : deprogram your subconscious mind, rewire the
 brain, and balance your energy / by RJ Spina.
Description: First edition. | Woodbury, MN : Llewellyn Worldwide ltd, 2023.
 | Includes bibliographical references. | Summary: "Using revolutionary
 teachings to help rewire your subconscious mind and bring balance to
 your energy, this book helps you finally be free of the stress, doubts,
 and low energy that block your joy and quality of life"-- Provided by
 publisher.
Identifiers: LCCN 2023006625 (print) | LCCN 2023006626 (ebook) | ISBN
 9780738774251 (paperback) | ISBN 9780738774367 (ebook)
Subjects: LCSH: Subconsciousness. | Mental healing. | Bioenergetics.
Classification: LCC BF315 .S63 2023 (print) | LCC BF315 (ebook) | DDC
 154.2--dc23/eng/20230614
LC record available at https://lccn.loc.gov/2023006625
LC ebook record available at https://lccn.loc.gov/2023006626

Llewellyn Worldwide Ltd. does not participate in, endorse, or have any authority or responsibility concerning private business transactions between our authors and the public.

All mail addressed to the author is forwarded but the publisher cannot, unless specifically instructed by the author, give out an address or phone number.

Any internet references contained in this work are current at publication time, but the publisher cannot guarantee that a specific location will continue to be maintained. Please refer to the publisher's website for links to authors' websites and other sources.

Llewellyn Publications
A Division of Llewellyn Worldwide Ltd.
2143 Wooddale Drive
Woodbury, MN 55125-2989
www.llewellyn.com

Printed in the United States of America

CHANGE
YOUR
MIND

Deprogram Your Subconscious Mind,
Rewire the Brain, and Balance Your Energy

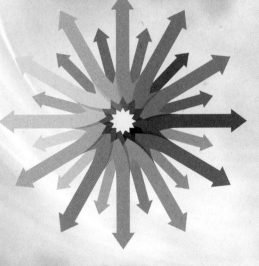

RJ SPINA

Author of *Supercharged Self-Healing*

Llewellyn Publications · Woodbury, Minnesota

Contents

Exercises

Disclaimer

The material in this book is not intended to be a substitute for trained medical or psychological advice. Readers are advised to consult their personal healthcare professionals regarding treatment. The publisher and the author assume no liability for any injuries caused to the reader that may result from the reader's use of the content contained herein and recommend common sense when contemplating the practices described in this work.

Dedication

This book is dedicated to all those who serve without seeking. May timeless truth, indomitable will, and unwavering compassion flow unabated through all humanity. May the wisdom, love, and power that we are created from be tangibly known within us all. May eternal divinity forever infuse the collective consciousness, transmute all disharmony, and remove the illusion of separateness. May the rising tide of timeless wisdom and unconditional love lift all ships and carry every Soul across hurricane waters.

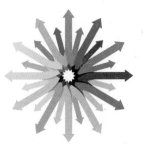

Introduction

Let me ask you a question: What would you be willing to do to be free of your constant stress, perpetual anxiety, ever-present doubt, and unsatisfying life? What if I told you there was a simple yet incredibly effective and mind-blowingly powerful way to change your mind and your life?

In today's chaotic world, did you know:

- 84 percent of adults in the United States report feeling stressed
- 47 percent suffer from anxiety
- 44 percent suffer from sadness
- 39 percent suffer from anger[1]
- 51 percent experience chronic fatigue
- 67 percent suffer from sleep issues
- Individuals under constant stress have a 50 percent higher mortality rate[2]
- Only 14 percent of Americans say they are happy ... the lowest in fifty years[3]

1. Bethune, "APA: U.S. Adults Report Highest Stress Level Since Early Days of the COVID-19 Pandemic."
2. Drah, "29 Disturbing Stress Statistics & Facts to Check Out in 2022," *Disturb Me Not* (blog).
3. Associated Press, "Americans Are the Unhappiest They've Been in 50 Years, Poll Finds."

This is the real global pandemic!

My friends, what would you be willing to let go of to feel powerful, truly alive, happy, and free? To be the limitless master you are that is temporarily housed within this biological garment we call a human being. Get ready, because you are about to discover how to uncover and then delete your subconscious programming that is exhausting you, stressing you out, and leaving you light-years behind your ultimate potential.

The key resides in your ability to make your limiting, Self-destructive subconscious programs visible to the conscious mind. These deep-rooted indentations and egoic identifications are what constrict your imagination and consume your energy. They prevent you from realizing your perfect, unlimited, and divine nature. They steal your precious life force and rob you of your potential, joy, peace, vitality, and loving nature.

Many of us have been programmed to endlessly torture ourselves by incessantly thinking (which locks us in time), over emotionalizing, and perpetually doing. Who and what have you really been obeying if you run yourself ragged to serve everything other than your own joy, peace, happiness, liberation, and spiritual evolution? For many, a patterned subconscious egoic mind robs us of tangibly knowing what we really are. Steady yourselves, my friends, for real magick is about to reveal it all!

The antidote to endless suffering is already within you. It is the awesome clarity, power, and freedom of the Real You! The Real You, or the Self, is not a who, per se. You are pure consciousness. More specifically, you are sentience given energy to create with. When you are in your normal, nonembodied, energetic state, you have no name or form. When incarnate, you remain a sentient wave of free, formless, unconditioned energy temporarily adorned with a human body.

There truly is no *who* to what you really are. It's all Source/God/Creator. There are, however, qualities and various amounts of this pure essence. At our core, we are love, wisdom, and power, whose subsets are talents and abilities. We are all made up of these universal characteristics. The more that you can accept and tangibly feel this truth, the greater your quality of life will be in every way.

Your Subconscious, Patterned, Egoic Mind Directs Your Every Behavior

Due to subconscious programming, many of us exhaust and delude ourselves in trying to "get things done." Eternal peace, ever-present completeness, unconditional love, and limitless imagination have been perverted and inverted into a low-frequency, programmed paradigm of endless duties and a worker bee mentality. When does it end and for whom? Both answers are the same illusion: your patterned, subconscious ego/mind/identity (EMI).

It is our energetic indentations and identifications (I am going to explain this in detail from a metaphysical perspective in chapter 1) of experiences, beliefs, concepts, traumas, expectations, ruminations, or even people that leave us perpetually imbalanced and drained. Our cravings and agonizing for satiation born from our patterned, subconscious, egoic mind cannot—and will never be—tangibly realized. You have been put under a spell. It only grows more and more powerful, draining your life force by the second the longer it goes unchecked!

Imagine finally being free of the stress, doubts, and low energy that prevent your true destiny, joy, and highest quality of life! The goal of this book and its teachings, exercises, and protocols is to change your mind and therefore your life. When we have a different understanding and we do different things, we get different results. A healed subconscious mind is the doorway to the stage of your infinite higher mind's potential to limitlessly play. All the world's a stage and, prior to reincarnating, you consciously choose this experience: the form factor (human vehicle), frequency (version of earth), script (life plan), and team (light or darkness). You are that powerful of a creator.

You are going to learn how to supercharge the process of deleting your hidden limitations to realize your power, freedom, peace, and joy! A truly awakened individual has no agenda except to experience the limitless depth and fullness of the Self. The joy and purpose of life itself will naturally and harmoniously flow through you but only if you learn to not mis-qualify your life force by allowing it to be consumed by your subconscious, patterned, egoic mind.

It is the embodiment of your subconscious, patterned, egoic mind—the false I—that blocks your highest potential and greatest joy. Once it does, the Real You has the experience of being confined, controlled, cornered, and constricted. I believe the most controlling and condescending people are those who are the most constricted and controlled by their subconscious, patterned, egoic mind. It can be no other way.

Your subconscious, patterned, egoic mind will rationalize everything it does. That is how it controls you and protects itself. Your finite mind/intellect is the justification for everything. There is no real acceptance, joy, completeness, forgiveness, freedom, or power at your disposal when you are operating under the spell of the patterned, subconscious, egoic mind. There is no unconditional love—for yourself or others—just appetite.

Get ready to discover for yourself how to deprogram your patterned, subconscious, egoic mind and meet the Real You. This challenge is twenty-one days long, and you will spend the first fourteen days doing your notebook exercise. The last seven days are to be spent running your energy diagnostic system. Remember, the difficulty or challenges you encounter are where your exponential growth resides. It's time to create a life befitting your limitless nature, unbreakable perfection, and eternal freedom.

The Directive Behind It All

Think of everything as a game for us to master ourselves as part of our endless spiritual growth. By design, our world culture celebrates egoic ideals, and we are conditioned to idolize those who personify them. This keeps our consciousness low frequency and therefore easily manipulated, led astray, and controlled. However, this also provides evolutionary tension. More evolved Souls use these examples of how not to be as an accelerant for their own evolution and ascension. Darkness, metaphysically speaking, always serves the light.

A fisher doesn't mind how many fish get away if they catch enough to fill their net. That is a way to understand the mindset of the low-frequency influence upon humanity. The low frequencies of the physical universe provide enough separation from where we come from and what we really are for this profound lack of Self-awareness to manifest. In other words, only in time/space can the experience of separation occur and therefore the very concept of relationships is born. The oneness has been lost. This is part of why the low frequencies are so difficult and offer such tremendous evolutionary opportunity.

In high-dive competitions, if you perform a very simple dive, like a swan dive, flawlessly, you still only receive a score of 7, maybe 7.5. But if you do a triple, 720 degrees, backward, spinning axle (you get the idea) and do it well, not flawlessly but well, you get a 9 or maybe a 9.5. Why? Degree of difficulty. The low frequencies—where we are right now—have the highest degree of difficulty and therefore they afford a Soul the greatest possible evolutionary content. You can very easily mess up those difficult dives as well.

Just for good measure, here's one more analogy! Think about high school; there is always a blend of freshmen, sophomores, juniors, and seniors. It's never all freshmen or all seniors. That would create an imbalance. There is—and therefore eternally must be—a balance and equilibrium to "what is." The same holds true on the deepest levels. We have a perfect balance of Souls on this planet for a safe and steady climb up the frequencies. Remember, the physical senses and intellect can never reveal the one true concrete reality. Think of it this way—we leave our journey here on the earth plane with a stronger back and a more tender heart. That is the very point and the literal evolution of our immortal consciousness.

Our Ancient Future of
Self-Transformation and Transcendence

Everyone has the capacity for total transformation. Absolutely everyone. I have seen it many, many times. We are an indirect fractal of God. No one lacks anything. Our repeated and cyclical physical incarnations are the miracle of alchemical magick born of higher-consciousness metaphysics.

What we are is sentience. The I AM. The kingdom of heaven lies within. Experiencing the infinite that is already contained within each one of us and bringing it out into physical manifestation is alchemy. The Source is within your consciousness. This wisdom captures the core of true alchemical Self-transformation.

Do not shy away from terms such as *magick*, *alchemy*, and *metaphysics*. We have all experienced supremely advanced civilizations on earth where these teachings and their teachers were part of our everyday existence. Higher-consciousness metaphysics, magick, and alchemy were an obvious part of our everyday lives just as brainwashing, censorship, cowardice, mind control, and pharmaceuticals are today.

Higher-consciousness metaphysics and true magick have been misappropriated, misused, and disguised by "leaders" for centuries against humanity. All of it is done for highly deceptive and nefarious purposes to distract, coerce, manipulate, subjugate, disarm, control, and destroy. In the deepest sense, the truth has been stolen from you. Not anymore, my friends.

The term *occult* or an *occultist* comes from the term *ocular* or an *oculist*, meaning "one who can see." All our understandings—be it science, religion, philosophy, physics, government, the arts—owe their origins to those who can see. Our entire world is based upon these teachings and understandings of the true teachers of humanity. They are known as the Ascended Masters.

About Me

Roughly seven years ago, I was told I only had forty-eight hours to live due to severe sepsis. I was "permanently" paralyzed from the chest down and riddled with chronic disease and other life-threatening conditions. Through my own authentic Self-realization, I remembered how Self-healing really works. I put my paralyzed and deathly ill body back together—just as I predicted I would in only one hundred days. The teachings and metaphysics I utilized became the foundation of my first best-selling book *Supercharged Self-Healing*.

Since that time, I have helped thousands of people all across the globe heal themselves mentally, emotionally, physically, and spiritually. The metaphysical, higher-consciousness protocols I teach awaken the direct connection to your own unlimited higher mind and free you from deeply rooted subconscious and egoic limitations. Through these enlightened metaphysics, humanity can experience a superior quality of life and accelerate its own ascension and spiritual evolution.

How to Use This Book

Change Your Mind is divided into three parts. In part 1, you will discover just how your entire behavior is dictated by a hidden aspect of yourself that the conscious mind has no direct access to … until now. You will discover the life-changing instructions for the revolutionary fourteen-day notebook exercise that literally brings your hidden and limiting subconscious programming into your conscious mind.

In part 2, the deprogramming of your subconscious, patterned, egoic mind allows a new awareness to emerge. Finally, you can meet the Real You that you always knew was inside, just waiting to break free of its limitations. With your new high-level access and understanding of the Real You, you will learn activities you can easily employ in your everyday life that seamlessly integrates the Real You.

In part 3, you will learn how to be expertly mindful of your most treasured resource: your energy. You will discover the revolutionary energy diagnostic system to manage and balance your energy bank account. You will have a quantifiable, repeatable, powerful, and effective way to measure and manage your energy.

You are about to discover how to finally illuminate your deep-rooted subconscious limiting programs. Once visible and tangibly understood by your conscious mind, you will never again be a prisoner to them! Let's get started!

Part 1

Understanding Your Subconscious Programming

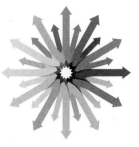

Chapter 1
What Is the Subconscious Mind?

Whatever you believe and think you are, that's what you're not.

The subconscious mind is a minor creation born of a loving, divine intelligence far beyond our human intellect. It's a creation of our Higher Self that allows it—and our Source—to both learn and concurrently experience through us. The subconscious mind is akin to the most highly sensitive recording and storage device imaginable.

It digitally and holographically imprints and records every single "now" you ever experience, including stimuli well beyond your physical sensory perceptions. This holds true not just regarding your current incarnation but every incarnation you've ever had or will experience, which are all happening right now! In essence, your entire body of multi-frequential energy, including your physical body, is the various recording energetic templates in which the subconscious mind is created by and for.

Our subconscious mind is not limited by the human brain. In actuality, the human brain is within and just an aspect of the far more voluminous and holistic subconscious mind. In our so-called waking state, we only have access to what I have termed the ego/mind/identity (EMI). Essentially, the EMI is the character your sentience creates through experiencing a low-frequency human incarnation.

Frequencies and the Self

Let's take a look at frequencies. A frequency is an assignation of energy. It is the rate at which energy vibrates within a specific environment. There is also dimension, which is a larger framework that houses frequencies. We don't exist dimensionally but rather frequentially.

Our Higher Self resides well outside of the physical universe, beyond space and time. It has no direct experience of the lower frequencies. It has no experience of what it's like to be cut off from Source/God/Creator, the Greater Reality. It knows nothing of the sensations of touch, taste, smell, low-frequency emotions, or physical sex. For it to learn what this slow, heavy, dense environment feels like, it must project a piece of itself—you—into this frequency, or "frequential environment."

For you to keep moving up the frequencies, you must evolve and master yourself—not the beliefs of the egoic identity—within every possible environment. This includes the lower frequencies of the physical universe where our version of earth resides.

Low-frequency disharmony cannot exist within a high-frequency environment. When we experience the lower frequencies of the physical universe, we lose direct access to the Self, or internal knowingness.

Your Subconscious, Patterned Mind

Because we drop down dimensionally and frequentially so drastically—as far as possible, actually—we lose understanding of what we really are and where we come from. It's like waking up at the bottom of the ocean with total amnesia while wearing a diving suit. This loss of holistic awareness and knowingness is so severe and total, we are left with beliefs. Because the energies are so dense here, we must temporarily merge and be housed within a biological garment (the human form) to exist here. Just like a diving suit or space suit.

This complete lack of Self-realization and access to where we come from creates a character—the ego/mind/identity—that we miscreate due to the electromagnetic interference of endless limited data we align ourselves with from this realm. It's not what you are, but instead it is a completely made up "who." Think of your human character as a shadow cast by the light inside you. Just like the shadows in Plato's cave, your shadow—and everyone else's—is simply a summation of your perceptions, understandings, and identifications. None—not one—are accurate, truthful, and authentic, and neither is your human character in comparison to what you really are.

What you are about to realize, among other hidden realizations revealed throughout this book, is that all your behavior is dictated by your subconscious, patterned mind. There is some overlap or cross-pollination with your egoic mind, and I will explain this in great detail shortly. Your so-called reality is created and constructed by your subconscious, patterned mind, not your conscious, thinking mind. Your conscious thoughts and emotions have little to no effect as they relate to the foundational underpinnings of your subconscious reality construction.

Your conscious, egoic mind (your EMI) is simply a low-frequency construct that loops the deeply embedded indentations of your subconscious programming. It keeps your patterned, subconscious mind perpetually hidden and increasingly dominant and therefore impossible to transcend.

But not anymore, my friends. There is an aspect of your higher mind that we can refer to as the super-consciousness. This super-consciousness is your Higher Self. I would not classify your higher mind as part of your subconscious mind but rather the other way around. Your subconscious mind is but an aspect of your higher mind.

For anyone who has read my first book, *Supercharged Self-Healing*, or watched some of my interviews, you know I love analogies. They are an essential medium that helps capture what we do not have the tangible experience nor understanding of. They are also a fun way to learn, which is why I like them! That being said, let's get right to a trifecta of analogies.

Bedspreads, Satellite Dishes, and Marbles

Imagine a very tight-fitting bedspread. Hospital corners, as they say. Now imagine placing a single marble somewhere on the bedspread. If we look closely, we can see that the marble has made a slight indentation upon the bedspread. Now imagine multiple bedspreads, stacked like a seven-layer cake, each one operating like a high-powered satellite dish, picking up various subtle waves of information (more marbles) and recording it all. All these bedspreads intermingle and inform one another.

Your multi-frequential body of energy, including your physical body (all of which is a projection from within your subconscious mind), is the layered bedspreads. A single marble is one solitary sensory perception that leaves an indentation upon the bedspread. Some of these sensory perceptions (marbles) can appear within the screen of your conscious mind and some are outside of it (beyond our physical sensory perception), yet they are still recorded and leave an indentation.

Every single thing you have ever seen, heard, smelled, tasted, or felt is a marble on your bedspread. Now think about all the stimuli that are outside your physical sensory perception, such as subliminal messaging, microwaves, X-rays, planetary forces, radio waves, cell tower frequencies, thoughts, emotions, desires, fears, etc.

Let's take it further (yes, more marbles!). Imagine all those marbles from thousands upon thousands of lifetimes and billions upon billions of parallel conditions. All that endless, incalculable, simultaneous, and concurrent experience. That, my friends, is a lot of marbles!

The marbles that heavily indent upon your multi-frequential bedspread of energy (which includes the physical body) are more like boulders. This could be anything from a traumatic event that you experienced to a story someone told you that shook you to your core. The bigger the marble, the bigger the indentation, and therefore the bigger impact upon your subconscious mind. The bigger the impact upon your subconscious mind, the bigger impact it has upon your behavior. Remember, none of these marbles are you.

What your conscious, thinking mind—"I"—is totally oblivious to is your entire thought/emotion processing and, subsequently, your actions and behaviors are perpetually and completely driven by these indentations. You, your conscious mind, is totally unaware and therefore not in control of any of it. You are going to discover this firsthand throughout this book as you learn how to deprogram your subconscious, patterned, egoic mind.

Subconscious Mind versus EMI

The main difference between your subconscious mind and your EMI are the conscious misidentifications you make. The totality of your limiting misidentifications forms your EMI. Your EMI is anything and everything you tack on to the statement I AM. I AM is the only statement you can ever make that is accurate, authentic, and eternally true. Everything after those two words is false.

This I AM is the indirect fractal of Source/God/Creator that you are in action. Pure, immortal, and untainted creator. I say indirect because we are roughly 2.5 percent of our Higher Self, or what I call our Totality. Your Higher Self, or Totality, is a direct creation of Source/God/Creator, and you are a projection (Soul) from your Higher Self—just like a tentacle is a smaller part of an octopus. I could tell you were needing another analogy, so there it is! Yes!

What you really are is immortal, formless, free, and unconditioned. You have no name, image, or identity. You lose all holistic awareness— inner Self-knowingness—due to the drastic and extreme fall in frequency upon incarnation into the physical universe. Because of this fall, you have replaced your deep knowingness and connectivity with beliefs/concepts/ideologies. These mental machinations (delusions) are the misperceptions, misunderstandings, and misidentifications that form your human character, your EMI.

Upon authentic Self-realization or enlightenment, these low-frequency temporary phenomena no longer cloud the truth. It is your dedication and devotion to inner silence and stillness—meditation—that removes the curtain of limiting Self-awareness and suffering. The exercises and teachings in this book will give you the tools to excavate what has been hidden by your own patterned, subconscious, egoic mind.

Here are a just few examples of conscious misidentifications we make that form our EMI human character:

- I am human/gender (misidentification with the physical body or form factor).
- I am a healer (misidentification with a talent, attribute, or quality).
- I am a banker (misidentification with a role).
- I am a certain religion (misidentification with a belief).
- I am a victim (misidentification with a limited, singular perspective).
- I am my thoughts (misidentification with mental machinations).
- I am my emotions (misidentification with the bathing of thoughts with energy).
- I am my past (misidentification with experience).

You are none of these things. You *create* them all. You are well beyond all of it and have existed before and after any of it. All the above statements are misidentifications with creations made by conscious choice. To be even more accurate, they are made through a non-Self-realized state of consciousness. This veil is what produces your misperception, misunderstanding, and misidentification with anything other than what you really are: I AM. Your EMI is the limitation program that runs by thinking...and you can only think in terms of what you have misidentified your immortal, free, formless, whole, complete, and unconditioned Self with.

Cross-Contamination of Subconscious Mind and EMI

The boulders that get embedded within your multi-frequential, layered bedspread of energy can become part of your EMI limitation program even without your conscious misidentification to it if there is significant enough impact/trauma upon your bedspread of energy. One example would be witnessing an emotional/mental/physical brutality that is traumatic enough to weigh upon your bedspread. The horror of war, murder, severe manipulation, torture, abuse, and gross injustice are enough to become part of the EMI even if it's not directed at you. Some things are such an affront to the vibration of love and wisdom—your essence—that you cannot process them in a depersonalized or detached way. Subsequently, they weigh upon you and become part of your EMI.

The other side of that coin is also true. For example, an act of unconditional love, benevolence, courage, and forgiveness can become part of your EMI. This may seem paradoxical because those are not traits of the EMI. They are closer to attributes of the True Self, or pure I AM. But if they become part of your false identity (EMI), they will be misappropriated and misused. Ultimately, even these purer attributes, once part of your EMI, will serve as a prison for your unlimited higher mind.

You can move forward with the understanding of the subconscious mind as being phenomena thrust upon, embedded in, and recorded within your multilayered bedspread that you don't have any conscious awareness of cocreating or identifying with. Conversely, your EMI are the phenomena you have consciously chosen to misidentify your nameless, pristine, divine, formless, free, and immortal essence with.

Summary

Just as the punch that we don't see coming always does the most damage, your subconscious, patterned mind has the biggest impact upon your every behavior. In fact, in a recent study neuroscientists have determined that 90 percent of reality creation comes from your subconscious mind.[4] Talk about massive unchartered terrain that simultaneously portends your limitless potential for exponential growth! This revolutionary book, and its enlightened teachings, will give you the keys to this previously hidden kingdom within us all. To live to your highest potential in every facet of your life, you must take what is buried within your subconscious mind and bring it into the light of your conscious mind. This is how you unearth and transcend all accepted forms of limitation.

In the next chapter, we are going to learn about the genesis of these revolutionary subconscious deprogramming teachings and how you can do them.

---

4. "How Your Subconscious Mind Creates Reality."

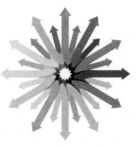

Chapter 2

Habits of the False Self

The Self, what you really are, is beyond all habits. It is an indomitable presence. Your essence has qualities, traits, and attributes, which we will get into later. Your human personality, which is created through incarnation into the lower frequencies of the physical universe (where you and I are now), is essentially a collection of habits born of subconscious programming and egoic identifications.

Think of most habits as the things you do unconsciously. Hence, they are products of subconscious programming. There is cross-pollination and a synergistic relationship with your EMI regarding this as well. There are many EMI habits you are completely conscious of, such as smoking, drinking, exercising, food choices, adhering to specific belief systems, capitulating to so-called authority, getting up early every day, what we choose to entertain ourselves with, etc.

Understanding the motivation behind your every desire, intention, thought, emotion, action, and behavior is power itself, and this clarity and liberation defeats all opponents, big or small. Living at the behest of your subconscious, programmed, egoic mind is the inversion and perversion of what you really are. It robs you of "what is"—your innate peace, completeness, divinity, freedom, and power to create without limitation.

Let's look at some universal habits we perform every day while under the spell of our patterned, subconscious, egoic programming and, most importantly, how to break them!

Spend as much time with each section until you feel a normalization of your new way of being.

Habit #1: Thinking

Thinking is simply the movement of the past; it's like mentally flipping through your Rolodex of memories (indentations and identifications). The past and future are just mental projections you habitually create rather than being fully present. Accept yourself completely, and you will simply be present.

Thinking is the rejection and nonacceptance of now. It is the reduction, fragmentation, compartmentalization, and contraction of Self—of life itself—through mentalization. Every thought you have had is not you, and it is impossible to experience and know the Real You through what you are not: thoughts.

By thinking, you trap yourself in the illusion of time. The past and future do not exist except in thought. Thinking creates the delusion of knowledge and the illusion of time. It's the main habit of humans, and its negative effect on your state of being and spiritual evolution is catastrophic.

Thinking is habitual and perpetual when you live in a reactionary state, and our reactions are the experience of our patterned, subconscious, egoic mind. Thinking is your looped program of marbles and boulders upon your energetic bedspread.

The patterned, subconscious, egoic mind hijacks your innate knowingness, love, and eternal freedom and replaces it with habitual, limiting, and predictive responses. At the top of the list is everybody's most overused program: thinking.

How to Stop Thinking

Pretend your two physical eyes are not attached to your brain. Or pretend you just arrived here—no past, no future. Or say, "I don't know, and I don't care."

If you do any of those three things, it should be impossible to think. Keep it up and watch how easily you overcome your lifelong subconscious habit of thinking. Remember, in pure observation action takes place. It is the activation of your divine intelligence, which has nothing to do with thinking. Thinking is a low-frequency side effect of subconscious programming and egoic identifications.

You will soon realize you can absolutely give up this limiting and low-frequency habit. Part of the subconscious mind operates like a storage device. We call this memory. It's one of the reasons why people undergo hypnosis and past-life regression. Your subconscious memorizes everything. You have absolutely nothing to think about. I will prove it to you.

Your entire life is memorized. You see a cup, and you know how to drink from it. You see a chair, and you know how to sit in it. You get in your car, and you know how to drive. You know how to wash, clothe, and feed yourself. You know where work is. You know where everything is in your house, where the store is, where your parents live, etc. Your entire life is memorized. You don't have anything to think about. Your subconscious mind has taken care of it for you.

Let's take the realization that you do not need to think even further. As you read this book, you understand every word without thinking. Sit with that for a moment. When you converse with someone, the same thing occurs. That's because real understanding—real communion with Self, one another, nature, your guides and helpers, even Source/God/Creator—only happens when you don't think.

Joy, happiness, love, and compassion occurs when you don't think. Your ascension, liberation, and infinite potential is only realized when you don't think. Conquer the habit of thinking and your life becomes yours once again.

Habit #2: (Mis)identifying

Misidentification occurs every time your patterned, subconscious, egoic mind has dominion over the eternal freedom of your higher mind. Anytime you see yourself as anything, such as the body/mind, gender, beliefs, roles, so-called knowledge (spiritual or otherwise), or experiences the body has, you are misidentifying. You are none of these things. You create them. You are pure awareness, not what you are aware of. You come way before all phenomena, and you are infinitely more than all of them put together.

Just as the clouds and bad weather never touch the sun, your misidentifications, no matter how severe or deep, never touch your essence. Misidentifications are temporary indentations upon your body of energy and/or attachments of your EMI. The Real You is unsullied awareness (two eyes floating with no brain attached) and forever untouched by it all.

The subconscious mind is "patterned" by its indentations. These patterns result in misidentifications, which dictate your predictive responses. Therefore, you recycle your experiences because your behavior is being driven by your patterned, subconscious, egoic mind. Without conscious access to the subconscious mind, we are compelled to react and behave in a limiting, inauthentic, and repetitive way.

Based upon what you now understand, see how easy and simple it is to control a population through subconscious programming. All you must do is engage in perception management, controlling what the five senses have access to, and those that have unconsciously acquiesced to their programmed, subconscious, egoic mind will simply, without questioning or fighting, do whatever they are told to do.

To liberate your mind, you must own your mind. Completely. Freedom is not doing whatever you want whenever you want. True freedom is escaping the tyranny of the mind. Once experienced, nothing can ever control you or hold you back.

How to Stop (Mis)identifying

Realize that whatever you can perceive, by definition, cannot be you. You are awareness itself, not what you are aware of. Never let that truth stop marinating within your heart. This defeats all programs of misidentification.

Habit #3: Reacting

The deliberate indentation upon your multilayered, energetic bed-spread is done to engender predictive and limited responses within a reactionary paradigm. Reacting to stimulus keeps you firmly within the parameters of your subconscious, patterned, egoic mind and therefore easily controllable.

Responding through detached observation awakens the Self directly. This activates your divine intelligence, which transcends all subconscious, egoic programming. Reacting and responding are opposites. Reacting is born of indentations and identifications (patterned mind), while responding (with unsullied perception and nonattachment) is born of a higher intelligence (the Self).

Reacting at the behest of your subconscious, patterned, egoic mind nullifies "what is," namely your natural ability to be fully present, compassionate, wise, and immensely powerful. Reacting is the experience of your subconscious programming having dominion over the complete majesty and infinitely spacious Self.

Remember, what you react to is your master. What you do not allow to simply come and go has usurped your inner completeness and peace. Reacting is not living. It's a total loss of Self-awareness and Self-control. Only the subconscious, patterned, egoic mind can have this effect upon your wholeness, love, divinity, power, and freedom.

How to Stop Reacting

Surrender to whatever appears within the screen of your consciousness. Meaning, don't immediately fight, analyze, or try to control. Simply surrender by giving yourself permission to be fully here, now, and the Real You will emerge.

Switch from the concept of acceptance to allowance. Acceptance locks you into "agreement" with one so-called reality. In other words, it is one way of perceiving things, therefore locking in a predetermined reaction based upon your programming. It limits you and pigeonholes the way in which you are perceiving.

Allowance keeps you open to the myriad ways of perceiving and experiencing and therefore unlocks you from programmed responses. It also allows for the transformation of what/who you are perceiving because it, too, is no longer locked within a set way from your programmed viewpoint.

Feel the difference within your body of energy when you say the word *acceptance*. There is a contraction. Now feel what happens when you say the word *allowance*. There is an expansion. This is tangible proof and the difference between the lower-consciousness programming and the infinite nature of the higher mind.

Habit #4: Needing to Be Productive

The Self—the Real You—is not programmed to constantly be doing something to be worthy or happy. The Real You is already whole and complete and does not quantify itself through the criteria of nonstop doing. That unholy directive is your conditioned, subconscious, egoic mind completely dictating your behavior.

The controller (subconscious, patterned, egoic mind) is controlled by indentations and identifications. This results in you being so completely and utterly controlled by these things that you are totally out of control. Always needing to be productive is born from a profound lack of Self-awareness, Self-acceptance, and Self-worth.

This specific subconscious programming relates to the production and consumption of physical goods. This way your frequency is kept low, and you automatically associate, limit, and misidentify yourself as a physical being. This inhibits your natural expansion of consciousness, a greater quality of life, and subsequent ascension up the frequencies. Quantifying your existence by needing to be productive is also part of the agreed upon "debt/slave reality," which is the very idea that everyone must work all day to pay for everything. The inception and conception of that belief system is a whole other conversation, my friends.

How to Stop Needing to Be Productive

Instead of measuring your day by how productive you've been, see how much presence (being-ness) you experience each moment. This is a true accomplishment. Gently and effortlessly bring your being-ness into your doing-ness by not mentalizing your every moment. When this becomes normalized, you are in the flow state. When doing becomes an effort, your subconscious, patterned, egoic mind has regained dominion of the Real You.

See yourself as a complete circle. There is nothing a circle needs. It is whole and complete as it is. The circle was designed to perpetually experience its own endless completeness and perfection. It never goes outside of itself because there is no need to. A circle is the primordial sacred geometric pattern in every way. So are you. Perfect in every way. Feel this.

Habit #5: Seeking Security

The subconscious, patterned, egoic mind is always in need of something (security and happiness) because it cannot experience eternal completeness. It's perpetually imbalanced. It's a pattern of indentations and identifications. It foments an impossible, unending quest trapped within limiting possibilities. This perpetually personalized and compartmentalized structure is what you call reality. Your personality is nothing more than your personal reality.

The subconscious, patterned, egoic mind, as we now know, is the energetic fabric upon which the indentations and identifications of sensory perceived data (and that which is beyond sensory perceived) are recorded and stored. To restore your bedspread to its original pristine state, you must protect/remove/release/repair all that is not germane to your original perfection.

You are constantly seeking the concept of security and the feeling of happiness. The idea that you (the body/mind) and what your character lays claim to ownership of (both tangible and intangible) are safe and protected is an illusion. Ownership does not exist. It's the product of a heavily conditioned and unawakened mind. Again, it's because you do not tangibly experience the ever-present fullness and happiness of the Real You.

The only real security is the Self. That is what a human being truly desires, and it can never be experienced through trying, seeking, or becoming. That's because you are already it. A dog doesn't have to try to be a do; it's a dog. You do not have to try to be yourself; you are the Self. Stop seeking security and watch what happens.

To dwell within as, for, and by the Self is the only true security. All things except the Real You—the Self—simply come and go, including this incarnation. Everything a human being does is always to preserve and secure its transitory existence and illusory identity. That behavior belongs to your subconscious, patterned, egoic mind.

How to Stop Seeking Security

Next time you sense your feckless and endless pursuit of never attainable security, stop and ask yourself, "Who is it that wants security?" Your answer will be, "Me, I'm the one who wants security." Then ask yourself, "Who am I?" The subconscious, patterned, egoic mind will go blank. That's because both the seeker and security are the same illusion. Both disappear under the simplest of scrutiny—and so does your suffering of them.

The only security that exists is the eternal and Immortal Self. Residing within and as the Self is the ultimate security. All seeking stops. You then realize you already are and have everything when you have the Self. You will also realize that no matter what you may lay claim to, you have absolutely nothing if you do not have your Self.

Habit #6: Craving Stimulation

Your inability to tolerate, let alone fall in love with, your own inner stillness, silence, and completeness is due to a lack of Self-awareness. Instead, you spend all your attention (and attention is energy, the very life force itself) under the spell of your subconscious programming. This manifests its sickness through your perpetual craving of stimulus simply to satiate and balance out the grooves of your patterned, subconscious, egoic mind.

Imagine your energetic bedspread with marbles and big rocks upon it. The craving of stimulus is you trying to compensate for those indentations and imbalances. Even the craving of so-called knowledge is the human character's foolish attempt to balance out its own total ignorance. Upon authentic enlightenment, both ignorance and knowledge are seen as the same thing and fall away. Watch your cravings, even for peace, and you will tangibly discover the truth about what drives the craving of any stimulation.

Subconscious cravings can run very deep. Sometimes oceans of time deep, assuming time authentically existed. It's all simultaneous experience; forget time. Think of space/time as a function of frequency rather than a concrete, fixed actuality. Craving stimulation only deepens and reinforces the subconscious and egoic programming. Satiating any craving only increases the imbalance. This creates a bigger and bigger subsequent craving, whose urge only increases in frequency and intensity.

How to Stop Craving Stimulation

Proper meditation gives you dominion over the mind/body complex. By having control over your energy, you gain control over all phenomena within your body of energy. This level of control stops further indentations/identifications and "smooths out" your energetic bedspread (patterned, egoic mind). Make the determination that you will never give in again to craving by harnessing your will so completely (having total control over your energy) that you become powerful beyond all measure. Mastery, my friends. It's your birth-right and destiny.

Here is an image for proper and powerful meditation to stop craving stimulation: imagine your head is a periscope, and the captain of the ship—the one looking through the periscope (you)—is deep within the hull, right in the center of your chest between your heart and spine. Never deviate from this and you will conquer your cravings.

Habit #7: Judgment

All judgment is Self-judgment and is based upon your patterned, subconscious, egoic mind. Judgment is the opposite of unconditional love, which is the one true concrete reality. When you judge anyone or anything, you are simply revealing your own conditioned mind. Judgment never affords you the experience of "what is."

Judgment is the inversion and perversion of love. When you judge, you are withholding your own equanimity and love from yourself. Rather than releasing/removing/repairing and forgiving yourself for your own imperfections, you opt for the easiest way out—the low-frequency habit of judgment.

Become aware of when you judge. Many "spiritual" people love to judge those they deem less awake and aware. It's their own egoic mind showing resentment for how they, too, were transfixed by the spell of their own subconscious, patterned mind. The patterned or unawakened mind expresses itself through resistance. Whatever triggers your judgment is your higher mind showing you where your indentations and identifications are still blocking your love.

How to Stop Judgment

The Self is so infinitely spacious that it has room for everyone and everything. Fully accept yourself, warts and all, and your judgment of yourself as well as "others" will stop. In truth, there are no others. We are just like the individual pieces of cookie dough placed on the cookie sheet; just moments before, they were all one. That's why all judgment is Self-judgment. See yourself in others. What harm can you do?

Realize that everyone, including yourself, is suffering. Everyone is going through something. Look into your own heart. Treat everyone with the same love, tenderness, and patience that you desire for yourself. Never forget what that nurturing feels like, and you will never judge again.

Habit #8: Chasing Pleasure

Chasing is behavior born of the concepts of incompleteness and lacking. Chasing is a disempowering experience brought on by the fractured, patterned mind. It illustrates a profound absence of gnosis or a tangible, experiential knowingness of the complete Self within.

The patterned, subconscious, egoic mind is always in need of something to balance its perpetual imbalance. This is the catalyst for greed. Whether it's mental, emotional, or physical, chasing pleasures belongs to the body/mind complex—not the Real You. Chasing is really an actor performing actions; the subconscious, patterned, egoic mind is the puppeteer and your body/mind complex is the puppet.

Know the truth: the desire you have for anything or anyone is really the desire to know yourself. Chasing pleasure is another example of trying to satiate what can never be satiated: desire. Giving in to pleasure only increases the attention we must give it each time. The pull and lure of the chase will only increase the attention/energy you give it. Attention is energy, and whatever you give energy to only increases.

How to Stop Chasing Pleasure

Experience every craving, in all its forms, as the captain way down inside the hull of the ship—right between the heart and the spine. This metaphysical truth will give greater "space" between sentience (you) and phenomena (body/mind).

Each craving is the ship's malfunctioning inner technology. Each time you refrain from altering your course by capitulating to pleasures, regardless of their severity, the ship corrects itself. It becomes sturdier and its functionality, performance, and durability improves. The voyage itself also gets calmer and more enjoyable.

Habit #9: Seeking Approval and Validation

As we strive to achieve a goal, we often tell people about it, announce it, or advertise it. Why? The subconscious, patterned, egoic mind is programmed to seek approval, validation, and reinforcement of its orders. The approval and validation are vital to satiate the subconscious with the concept of "success." Without it, along with the continuous reinforcement, the hold or effectiveness of the brainwashing wanes.

Once the higher mind begins to unfold through the teachings and exercises within this book, you are empowered rather than programmed to mindlessly perform tasks to achieve and become. This is the difference between reacting and responding. Reacting is disempowering, while responding through conscious choice is empowering. To have your life be truly your own, you must take the mind back first.

How to Stop Seeking Approval and Validation

Seeking approval is simply a low-frequency commiseration (group think) and validation is a permission slip (seeking empowerment from a disempowered state) to continue or pursue a specific behavior. Instead, realize the truth: if your endeavor requires outside approval or validation, this notion is not authentically yours to begin with.

Before impulsively and mindlessly obeying your subconscious programming to seek approval and validation, stop. Instead, simply pretend you just arrived here—no past or future. Stay that way, fully here, now, until you tangibly feel your own towering and monumental presence consume the patterned, subconscious, egoic mind.

Habit #10: Asking for Permission

The Real You—the Self—is completely and utterly free. It is not impelled or compelled to ask for permission from anyone for anything. Ever. Asking for permission is what the subconscious, patterned, egoic mind does because it lacks any true authenticity and therefore has no real power to act on its own authority.

Asking for permission is birthed from a programmed state of disempowerment. Who is the one asking for permission? It can only be an actor (not the Real You) performing an action (not of your own accord). See the habit of asking for permission for what it really is: the subconscious, patterned, egoic mind living in a programmed, disempowered, and inauthentic state.

The subconscious, patterned, egoic, mind has no tangible experience of authentic freedom or true power. Only a brainwashed individual (prisoner) trapped within its own disempowering limitations seeks permission to continue living within its own Self-imposed jail.

How to Stop Seeking Permission

Mantra:
"My power and independence rise,
My I AM roars; no more disguise!"

Repeat that mantra either out loud or utilizing the silently spoken word until its full power and depth of transformation is a tangible reality for you.

You are an immortal and limitless creator being. You exist to create like the limitless master that you are. Permission is absolute and without question. Your proof is the very life force itself that eternally flows through you. There is your permission and your proof.

Habit #11: Needing Attention

You seek attention because you are disconnected from the completeness of the Real You or Self. Only the subconscious patterned egoic mind "thinks" or "feels" it needs anything. It is compelled to obey its programming of unworthiness and incompleteness. It always needs something in subservience to its programming.

Attention is energy, and that's why the patterned, subconscious, egoic identity seeks attention, namely from you. Without it, the patterned mind stops having sway over you. What you are not—the patterned, subconscious, egoic identity—seeks attention, craves achievement, and tries to become, all of which are the opposite of "what is." Your direct, tangible experience of the eternal and inherent completeness within—the Real You—is "what is."

Needing attention only temporarily fills and engages that which is eternally imbalanced: your subconscious, patterned, egoic mind. This imbalance only increases its energetic demands on you and others the more you obey it. Needing and getting attention doesn't end the craving for attention; it feeds it.

How to Stop Needing Attention

Like water draining from a bathtub, let all the energy drop down out of your mental body (head) and emotional body (solar plexus). Continue to let it drain down until all your energy gently sits just beneath the belly button and above the groin. Now recognize that your mind has become completely clear and your emotions have totally stabilized.

Now use your eyes as if there is no brain attached to them and just be pure awareness. Anytime the need for attention is recognized, repeat this process. Soon enough, you will defeat the patterned, subconscious, egoic mind's program of needing attention.

Habit #12: Needing to Be Right

Needing to be right is a favorite and horrifyingly debilitating pastime of the subconscious mind and EMI. The Real You is constantly unfolding and learning about itself. The patterned, subconscious mind and EMI stop the evolution of your consciousness by refusing to be open-minded and thus evolve. Needing to be right only recognizes personalized indentations and identifications. The subconscious, patterned mind and EMI will defend them to the death because it sees itself as them.

Examine the need to be right and how it is born of a fear-based reactionary state for control. This need for control is birthed to make sure "reality" coincides with the subconscious, patterned, egoic mind. Without exerting control due to the need to be right, the programming and false identity falls apart. Watch how you get triggered when "what is" doesn't align with your subconscious, patterned, egoic identity.

Needing to be right is one of the more deadly pastimes, which you must avoid at all costs. This need to be right stops your evolution. The unfurling and expansion of consciousness has ceased. This is called disinformation in today's world, but it's really the fear of dissent. From a metaphysical perspective, needing to be right promotes stagnation, which engenders degradation, followed by demise. If you are not evolving, there is no longer any point in being here. The universe Self-directs, Self-corrects, and Self-evolves—always.

How to Stop Needing to Be Right

When the urge to control and be right is recognized, just stop and surrender to the idea that your understanding of things is merely a single opinion within a sea of eight billion opinions. None of those opinions are "what is" but rather an infinitesimally limited interpretation. That's it.

Do not hide, take solace, or gain comfort from group think. Capitulating to any agreed upon version of a co-opted reality only suits further servitude to your subconscious, patterned egoic, mind and the tyranny it breeds.

Summary

Whatever we are the awareness of—including the awareness of awareness itself—is nothing to give any real gravitas to. It will all come and go. Most of us associate fighting and overcoming challenges and injustice as the triumph of the will. It certainly can be, without question.

However, at a certain point in your own evolution, surrender is the highest use of your will. Gently use your will to stop fighting yourself. Stop trying to control, to be right, to be productive. Stop trying to ward off fear by hanging on to beliefs, concepts, thoughts, sensations, people, and things. Just stop fighting your own shadow.

Surrender to the exquisite symphony of silence, the never stagnant nor stationary perpetual vibration of pristine inner stillness. The majestic and seemingly empty yet total completeness of the immortal, divine, and unconditioned Self will be tangibly known. That's the Real You.

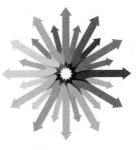

Chapter 3
Starting to Deprogram
the Subconscious Mind

When your attention is upon thoughts/emotions/bodily sensations, you are giving them energy. Attention is energy. The story of "I"—the egoic voice inside your head—is continually being fed, kept alive, and grown by your attention to it. This only results in your experience of greater separation from Self, increased disharmony, and seemingly concrete limitation.

What is happening is that you are getting further and further from the tangible truth about what you really are. This abyss between gnosis (Self-knowledge) and illusion is created because of a lack of tangible Self-awareness and its ever-present dance partner: no Self-control. Therefore, you do not experience total freedom, Self-contained completeness, unbreakable inner resolve, and limitlessness creativity.

Accept yourself fully, warts and all, and you will effortlessly be present all the time. You will cease to be held back by your own subconscious programming and egoic limitation program. You will begin to experience the completeness and limitless depth of yourself. The divinity, awe, and richness inherent within every moment will carry you across hurricane waters. The tangible experience of the infinite possibilities inherent within each moment is your playground now and forever.

How to Experience Liberation and Freedom

Roughly fifteen years ago, my desire to liberate myself from the human character called RJ consumed me. I could not see my subconscious programming, but I certainly felt it. It was dictating my every behavior and every thought. All I was experiencing was my subconscious programming and not me directly. I was compelled to undo all that was holding me back. I knew—I could feel it in my blood—that my mind was trapped within a maze of beliefs, indentations, and identifications. Unfortunately, I could not see them clearly enough to eradicate them.

I said to myself that I must destroy everything about RJ that was not authentically and directly my essence. I was willing to lose everything because I didn't fully have myself. Therefore, I had nothing. I was willing to experience physical death to be truly free, but I knew testing the limits of my body wouldn't do it. (My potentially lethal sepsis, "permanent" paralysis, chronic disease, and life-threatening conditions would challenge me many years later!) Instead of experiencing death, here's what I did…

My first order of business was to buy a new notebook and a pen. I then took two weeks off from work. I intuitively knew that to deprogram my subconscious, patterned mind, I needed to consciously see and tangibly understand my motivation behind my every notion, so I wrote everything down that I was doing. Everything. Every notion, thought, action, and behavior. I mean *everything*. I needed to write it all down so I could see it consciously. Then I preceded to relentlessly question and demand to know the core motivation driving my every behavior.

I knew in my core that until I could see why the character RJ was the way he was, I would never be able to transcend his limitations. I demanded my own liberation and decided I would stop at nothing—I mean nothing—to experience my total freedom and Self-realization.

What I discovered was an incredibly simple yet mind-bogglingly effective protocol. Inherent within the simplicity of Self-inquiry is the elegance of total clarity and the power of complete transformation.

I knew I needed to tangibly see and realize what I AM. Once known, everything else would fall away. I could feel that I was thinking/emoting/acting/behaving from things already implanted, a place before my conscious mind. These indentations upon my brain, body, and body of energy—along with the misidentifications I consciously chose (EMI)—needed to be revealed and seen by my conscious waking mind. I had to go deep within the recesses of my subconscious mind to discover and experience what I AM before any of this.

Change Your Mind:
Life-Changing 14-Day Notebook Exercise

Get yourself a small notebook/journal and a pen. Always keep your notebook/journal and pen with you. I do not suggest a computer for this exercise. If you can take time off from work, as I did, I highly recommend it. When you do have a day off from work, do this exercise all day. Each time you reach out to text, email, or call someone, turn on the TV, scroll social media, look up information, go shopping, you name it, question it! Uncover the real motivation behind your actions and behaviors. You won't believe what you discover about yourself!

If you must work, do this exercise upon waking until your workday starts and then resume it after work is completed up until bedtime. If you can "notebook" during work, do it. This exercise will continue to peel the onion of your patterned, subconscious mind, which includes your work life, like nothing else. You are going to use your journal/notebook like an archaeologist would use their shovel to unearth what originally existed buried beneath the layers of rubble and time.

The first morning of your fourteen-day challenge, once you catch yourself performing any action, thought pattern, or behavior, stop, and write it down. Then question it until you get to the core motivation driving your behavior.

Here is the very first example from one of my notebooks that I have kept all these years.

Example #1: Notebook Exercise

Upon awakening the very first morning of my notebook exercise, I found myself needing to go to the bathroom. As I entered the bathroom, I caught a glimpse of my unkempt hair in the bathroom mirror. Reflexively I reached for my hairbrush and began to brush my hair. Before I realized it, I was already mindlessly performing an action, so I abruptly stopped.

The following is taken directly from my personal notebook:

> **BRUSHING MY HAIR.**
> *Question:* Why I am brushing my hair?
> *Answer:* So it looks good.
> *Question:* Why do I care if my hair looks good?
> *Answer:* So other people find me attractive.
> *Question:* Why do I care if other people find me attractive?
> *Answer:* Because I get a sense of my own Self-worth based upon other people's opinion of me.

My jaw dropped. This discovery was revelatory! It felt like my head was just split open. The true motivation behind brushing my hair was completely driven by other people's opinions of me. It was 100 percent my subconscious programming that became part of my EMI. I felt freer and empowered the very instant this epiphany washed over me.

Other people's reactions and opinions regarding you say everything about them and nothing about you. Judgment says everything about the one doing the judging and nothing about what is being judged. My first questioned behavior revealed to me that I didn't know myself. Instead, I was programmed to rely upon judgment and societal pressures to get a sense of myself. In that moment, I tangibly realized that only I define me (limit myself or not). This was true empowerment beyond all measure.

You are about to do the exact same thing for yourself! All by simply writing down your actions/behaviors and getting to the true motivation behind what is driving them. This work is real magick because it completely reveals what has been hidden (your subconscious programming) and helps make it disappear. Merlin the Great would be proud of you!

Being brutally honest with myself gave me a clear landscape of my subconscious, patterned, egoic mind. Only upon "seeing" what my true motivation was behind brushing my hair could I break that spell/habit—if I chose to. That spell/habit was in control of my behavior, and spells/habits are manifestations of the past. Now when I brush my hair, it's not an action driven by anything other than conscious creative choice. That is power.

Imagine, all these life-changing revelations from just the understanding of why I really brush my hair! This was the very first behavior I performed on the first morning of my notebook challenge. I have three notebooks filled with these life-altering epiphanies. By the time I was done with my notebook exercise challenge, I had never felt freer, happier, more confident, more powerful, and more like my Self in my entire life.

On the surface, it may seem extreme to question everything one does to this degree. Perhaps it is, but I will say this: Not questioning and truly understanding why you operate the way you do is a pointless and crushing existence. It is guaranteed to leave you controlled, cowardly, confined, complicit, and constricted in this life. You deserve far more, my friends. Now, with these teachings, create a life—your life—befitting what you really are. A life filled with truth, purpose, love, meaning, joy, power, and passion (just to name a few)!

The very point of existence is for it to know itself in totality. Not investigating yourself gently and relentlessly is contrary to the very mandate of all existence. It is my Soul's primary desire to offer these

Self-realized understandings so you can uncover the Real You and usher in a new way of being on this planet!

Example #1: Notebook Exercise Deconstructed

Let's do a quick review and deeper dive into my hair-brushing example.

First, write down your action/behavior. Brushing my hair. Then, ask yourself, "Why am I doing this action/behavior?"

> *Question:* Why am I brushing my hair?
>
> *Answer:* So it looks good.

The first answer will be a justification, not the core motivation. Once you get your initial response, ask yourself again, "Why do I feel or care or think that way?" You will get another answer, but it won't be your core motivation.

> *Question:* Why do I care if my hair looks good?
>
> *Answer:* So other people find me attractive.

You are getting closer to your subconscious and/or egoic programming. At this point, your continued questioning and truthful answers are where the transformation takes place. Keep asking yourself, as I did, until you get to the core, original motivation behind the action or behavior.

> *Question:* Why do I care if other people find me
>   attractive?
>
> *Answer:* Because I get a sense of my own Self-worth
>   based upon other people's opinions of me.

This reveal is true magick because it provides authentic alchemical transmutation and transformation! My motivation for performing that action was due to societal conditioning and egoic gratification.

It is only once you stop living and behaving for things buried within your patterned, subconscious, egoic mind that you will ever really know the beauty, joy, freedom, completeness, and limitless nature of the Real You. Do this life-changing, transforming note-book challenge and your life will never be the same because by the time you are done, it will finally and truly be *your* life!

Example #2: Notebook Exercise

A few days into my notebook exercise, I found myself reaching for my phone to text message a friend of mine. I immediately grabbed my notebook. Remember that honesty, courage, and discipline are the key. I wrote down:

> TEXT MESSAGING MY FRIEND.
>
> *Question:* Why am I text messaging my friend?
>
> *Answer:* To see how he is doing.
>
> *Question:* Do I really want to see how he is doing?
>
> *Answer:* No, not really.
>
> *Question:* Then why am I really text messaging him?
>
> *Answer:* I feel lonely.

Now I was really getting somewhere. I could feel it. I knew if I was courageous and honest enough with myself, I would uncover what I needed to see.

> *Question:* Why do I feel lonely?
>
> *Answer:* I want attention.
>
> *Question:* Why do I want attention?
>
> *Answer:* Because I don't know what to do with myself.
>
> *Question:* Why don't I know what to do with myself?
>
> *Answer:* Because I don't know myself. I can't tolerate my
>   own inner stillness and silence.

Something shifted in me. I felt like something was being lifted off me. I felt lighter. Happier. In that moment, because I was honest with myself, I was able to accept myself like never before in my life.

Example #3: Notebook Exercise

I had just got off the phone with a family member. I realized something profound the moment the conversation had ended: I needed to be right. I wrote:

> **BEING RIGHT.**
> *Question:* Why do I need to be right?
> *Answer:* Because I want people to know the truth.
> *Question:* The truth about what?
> *Answer:* Whatever we are talking about it.
> *Question:* Do I really care if people know the truth?
> *Answer:* No, I just want people to know how smart I am.

Again, with courage and honesty, real transformation can take place.

I kept questioning myself. Below is an example of both subconscious and EMI programming.

> *Question:* Why do I care if people think I am smart?
> *Answer:* Because it makes me feel good about myself. I identify with being smarter than everyone. It's vanity.
> *Question:* Why do I bother with vanity?

The next moment was a question and answer simultaneously…

> *Answer/Question:* Because without it, what do I have?
> *Answer:* My Self. Peace. My own contentment and happiness.

I could not believe what just hit me. In that moment, I realized I was the one keeping myself from myself. It was me! I was too busy focusing on my vanity. Being right, being smart, being seen by others as highly intelligent. I wasn't enough for myself because I really didn't have myself.

I needed others to see me a certain way to reinforce my subconscious programming, my EMI, my false identity. I had traded the compulsion to be right with the ability to be content with myself. I exchanged needing validation with being at peace. I bartered away my own happiness and completeness in exchange for seeking something from others.

My inner world shifted yet again. I was beginning to see how everything I was doing was at the behest of my subconscious, patterned, egoic mind. All of it. This notebook exercise was liberating me from everything that caused my experience of lacking, stress, suffering, anger, and worry.

The more I continued with the notebook exercise, more aspects of my life that weren't serving my liberation left me. I no longer felt stress or frustration. I began to feel freer and lighter. I had more energy, happiness, and peace. I felt more like my Self and more powerful than ever before!

Now, it's your turn. Follow exactly as I have outlined for you. Be brave. Be honest. Be what you really are. You are worth every moment of excavation to discover the Real You.

More Notebook Exercise Examples

If you are struggling with this exercise, perhaps it will help to see more examples. I have helped many people work through the notebook exercise over the years. Here are a few examples that show how the exercises have helped my clients release their EMI.

Rebecca

Rebecca is a massage therapist and Reiki master in her late thirties. She lives in her new condo in downtown Phoenix, Arizona. She is smart, articulate, and sensitive, enjoys what she does, and takes care of herself physically and financially.

If we judged a book by its cover, we would all assume Rebecca is leading the perfect life, but the physical senses can never reveal the one true concrete reality. During our first remote session, Rebecca began by telling me how evolved she is and how together her life was.

"I received my massage license about two years ago. It's going great. Lots of repeat clients. I'm not taking on any new clients; I'm so busy."

"That's fantastic. I'm happy to hear that."

"I started doing Reiki about eight years ago. I love energy work too. I find I can really connect with people's energy whether doing Reiki or massage. I'm good at both."

Her voice started to trail away as she finished her last sentence. Intuitively, I already felt she was hurting beneath that wonderful facade. I held a high frequency for her so she had the space to be honest with me and, more importantly, with herself.

"I'm sure you are, Rebecca. Would you like to tell me what's troubling you?"

I could feel the swell of her emotions surging through her. She tried to keep a lid on it by clamping it all down.

"It's okay. It's okay," I said.

With permission to let go, the dam broke and so did her facade. I kept my focus on what she really is—divinity incarnate—and that helped maintain the high frequency and the space she needed to heal.

"Just leave everything here with me," I told her.

As Rebecca sobbed, her shoulders shuddered, and her breath came in spurts. We said nothing for at least thirty seconds. There was no need. What was being communicated and shared—her pain and my compassion—was well beyond words. Eventually she began to regain control of herself as she wiped away her tears.

"RJ, my intimate relationships always leave me totally defeated and drained. Every single time. I feel broken, used up, and hollow. My heart and my mind can't take it anymore. It's making me physically sick. I don't know what to do anymore."

Now that it was out in the open, we could begin uncovering the root cause of her suffering: the subconscious, patterned, egoic mind.

She went on, "Every guy I get involved with, it's the same story. I give and give, and they take and take. And I can never make it work. I am never going to be happy."

"Rebecca, until you see and understand what is driving your behavior, you can only recycle your experiences."

That seemed to catch her attention.

"Nobody is broken. What you are is untouched—just like the sun is untouched by the bad weather. What you really are is unscathed by whatever goes on with the body/mind."

The truth was tangibly registering within her. Her breathing stabilized, and her eyes became clear as I went on.

"The program your subconscious mind is running doesn't work because the Real You, what you really are, is already whole, perfect, and complete. That's why you can't handle such imperfection, courtesy of your subconscious, patterned, egoic mind, anymore."

The pain and sorrow that was emanating from Rebecca's azure-colored eyes ceased. Calmness and clarity were taking over because Self-recognition was occurring. The seeds of liberation had taken root. I explained to her the notebook exercise and suggested she give it 100 percent effort over the next two weeks. She said she would do it, and we agreed to have another session at that time.

Two weeks later, it was time to start my workday. For me, that includes a coffee. Ever since I got my own espresso machine, I have become horribly spoiled by delicious homemade java. Today I went with an organic double espresso from Peru mixed with oat milk and a touch of whip cream. Now I was ready to work!

I flipped open my day planner, logged on to my computer, and opened my virtual meetings for the day. I clicked on my first scheduled appointment. Rebecca was already waiting.

"Hi, Rebecca. You are absolutely glowing."

"I feel like a phoenix risen from the ashes."

"Fantastic. Please tell me everything."

"RJ, first off, I have never felt this way in my entire life. I feel light, free. I am truly happy. I can't believe it. Can I read something to you?"

"Of course."

"This is from the notebook exercise I wrote down."

TEXT MESSAGING MY BOYFRIEND AT WORK.

Question: Why am I checking in to see how my boyfriend is feeling?

Answer: Because I feel responsible for his happiness.

Question: Why do I feel responsible for his happiness?

Answer: Because it's my job to make sure he is happy.

Question: Why do I feel it's my job to make sure he is happy?

Answer: Because I don't want to fail.

Question: Why do I think I failed if someone else isn't happy?

Answer: Because it means I'm not good enough.

Question: Not good enough for what?

Answer: For anybody. I don't deserve to be in a relationship if I can't make someone happy. I'm not good enough. I need to make someone else happy so I feel better about myself.

Rebecca continued, "RJ, I finally realized my subconscious pattern of trying to make other people happy was because of a lack of Self-worth. I've been a people pleaser my entire life. In every relationship—friends, my parents, boyfriends. Now I know why. I don't value myself, so I constantly focus on others."

"This is an amazing insight, Rebecca."

"I never felt comfortable in my own skin. So instead of accepting and loving myself, I would just focus on making sure everyone else was happy. In fact, I would learn and then obsess over what I could do to help, fix, or please them! Therefore, I always felt empty, used up, and unfulfilled every time—in every relationship."

I was so proud of her, and the huge smile across my face made it obvious.

Rebecca was so excited she continued, "The moment I saw in black and white that I always put my desire to please others ahead of my own well-being and happiness, it shifted. I totally get it now. I kept having the same heartbreaking experience over and over in all my relationships. Even with my parents and friends. I kept trying to help others and fix everyone. Now I realize I couldn't break that pattern because I never saw why I was really doing it."

"Helping, fixing, and serving are three very different ways of seeing life. When you help, it's because you have a very deep-rooted belief that life is weak. When you fix, it's because you have a deep-rooted belief that life is broken. When you serve, you see life as whole and complete. Fixing and helping are subconscious, egoic programs. They are draining and onerous. They have a very tangible energetic quality to them. Service feels completely different. It effortlessly flows from the Self. It never wanes. Feel it. Being in service has a completely different energetic quality than helping or fixing."

"Oh my God. You're so right. Helping and fixing is exhausting. Serving is more like sharing and doesn't drain you."

"Precisely. Because being of service comes from the one true unending source: the Self."

Rebecca is a completely different person now that she is deprogramming her subconscious, patterned, egoic mind. She is living a life of greater authenticity and clarity. Her energy level is through the roof, and she feels more at peace and happy with herself for the first time in her life. That's because she finally knows her True Self. Bravo, Rebecca!

Gary

Gary is in his mid-forties and lives in Denver, Colorado. He owns multiple small businesses and is always on the go. He is physically fit, tan, and presents a neat appearance. Gary was visiting his elderly mom in San Diego. He read my first book and decided it was the time to connect with me.

In his initial visit to my office, he requested help and guidance regarding OCD and business success. My assistant told him we could address his concerns in our session. Gary booked the first open appointment with me the following month. The timing was perfect because he was attending a conference that evening in the local business district where my office is.

Gary arrived all smiles, dapper, and quite eager. Intuitively it was obvious to me he used his charm and high energy to get what he wanted in life. I met his gaze as we shook hands, and I offered him a seat. I took a sip of my hazelnut-flavored espresso with almond milk and settled into my chair.

"Nice to see you, Gary. What would you like to discuss today?"

"RJ, I work hard, too hard, but I never seem to get any real traction with what I am doing. I have three businesses and have been trying to build each one for a few years, but I don't have anything to really show for all the effort I put in."

"In what way? Monetarily? Inner fulfillment? Purpose? Or all three?"

"All three. I don't understand why they all seem to fail. I just feel stuck. I'm spinning my wheels and only getting more compulsive and anxious about everything by the minute. I'm not young anymore, and I don't want to keep failing. I should have more at this stage of my life." Gary rubbed the back of his neck to try and soothe himself. He looked down at his shoes, lips pursed, and shook his head in bitter disappointment.

"Until we understand what is truly driving our behavior, we can only recycle our experiences."

"What do you mean?"

"Our subconscious mind creates our reality and dictates our every behavior. We don't realize this because we do not have access to our subconscious mind. Most human beings focus on results rather than the understanding of the core motivations driving their desire in terms of the life they are trying to build. This hidden motivation expresses itself as our day-to-day behavior. Until we see what is bathed in darkness—the subconscious, patterned, egoic mind—we can only recycle our experiences and thus, keep manifesting the same limiting results."

This understanding left Gary speechless. He began to look around my office as his mind searched for a solution. He finally brought his eyes back to mine.

"Can you help me?"

I let the question hang for a second.

"I can show you exactly what to do…only if you promise to see the entire process through."

"I promise."

"No."

My eyes, serious as a sheet of flame, zeroed in on his. As I spoke, each word was imbued with the vibration of unbreakable will.

"Not to me. Promise yourself. Make the commitment right now, to yourself, that you will never let yourself down again."

Gary's eyes widened. The energy was palpable. He was being shifted. It reminded him of what was buried inside of him—inside all of us.

"I'll do it. No matter what."

With that, a tear of fierce determination streamed down his right cheek. His faith and will had been reawakened. I smiled and gently nodded in agreement.

"Yes, you will."

I shared with Gary how to deprogram his subconscious mind using the notebook exercise. I gave him specific examples from my personal notebook. I told him that through true dedication, courage, and honesty, that in just a few weeks, his life will not only radically change and improve, but for the first time, it will truly be his life.

Two weeks later for our next session, I decided to meet Gray at beautiful Coronado Beach by the famous Hotel del Coronado and at the very end of the eastern side of it is a dog beach section. My best friend, Marlon, a Jack Russell Chihuahua mix, left his body in August 2020. This beach was his favorite place in the world besides my lap, and his ashes were scattered precisely where I stood.

I turned around and saw Gary. With a notebook in hand, he was excitedly slogging his way through the hot, dry sand to meet me at the water's edge. Not even the slightest bit out of breath upon arrival, Gary bowed to me, smiling from ear to ear.

"I'm a new man, RJ. I have never felt this free or this empowered in my entire life."

"It warms my heart to hear you say that. I'd love to hear what you learned."

As warm, foamy waves lapped our toes, Gary proudly flipped open his journal and pointed to this specific passage:

> IN A RUSH TO HAVE BREAKFAST.
>
> *Question:* Why am I in a rush?
>
> *Answer:* Because I always have a lot to do.
>
> *Question:* Why do I always feel I have a lot to do?
>
> *Answer:* Because my life will fall apart if I don't rush.
>
> *Question:* Why do I feel like my life will fall apart if I don't rush?
>
> *Answer:* Because I need to control everything to keep it going.
>
> *Question:* Why do I feel I need to constantly control everything if it's not working anyway?
>
> *Answer:* Because I don't want to fail.
>
> *Question:* Why am I afraid to fail?
>
> *Answer:* Because I need to succeed.
>
> *Question:* Why do I need to succeed?
>
> *Answer:* I need it to feel good about myself.
>
> *Question:* Why do I not feel good about myself right now?
>
> *Answer:* I don't like who I am. I'm not good enough.
>
> *Question:* Not good enough for who?
>
> *Answer:* For me. I try to control everything by working too much because I don't like how I feel about myself. I don't want to feel this way, so I work like crazy to

feel better about myself. Deep down, I don't like myself or trust that I'm good enough. And that's why everything always fails.

And then he showed me another section.

CRYING.

Question: Why am I crying?

Answer: Because this horrible feeling about myself that I have had since I was a kid is finally leaving me.

Gary turned to me and smiled as dogs barked and played in the water.

"This is amazing, Gary."

"RJ, the moment I wrote an answer down, it's like I immediately started feeling free of it. Once I could see it, really see it, I didn't have to let it consume me anymore. It's just like it was all being pulled right back out to sea ... and I was free."

I was so proud of him. There was nothing I felt compelled to add, but Gary wasn't done.

"About five days into the notebook exercise, I started to feel so much better. I felt more spacious inside. Lighter. Happier. About a week later, all my businesses started to pick up a bit. Not a lot but noticeably. I wasn't even trying as hard as before. It's like I could breathe better, and my businesses expanded."

"You changed your understanding of yourself through the work you just did. That new understanding changed your vibration. Your vibration is what the universe mirrors back in what we call manifestation. You did it with less effort and angst by raising your vibration."

Through the notebook exercise, Gary brought his subconscious programming into his conscious mind and subsequently changed his life. He is now empowered and feeling worthy as he is. He now feels that the Real Him is in conscious control of his thoughts, actions, and behaviors.

His newfound well-being and Self-worth have directly translated into a significant increase in material success. Previously Gary's inability to feel capable of powerful "positive" manifestation had been subverted by the subconscious programming of no Self-worth and no Self-confidence. Now, Gary lives empowered and more peacefully through his higher-frequency state of being, and his entire life reflects that.

Sarah

I met Sarah a few months ago. We were both traveling to visit family. Sarah is in her early forties, quick witted, and lives in Sioux Falls, South Dakota. She is a registered nurse practitioner and an avid jewelry maker.

Upon our random meeting, Sarah was immediately and sincerely interested in the healing I experienced. She was also fascinated with the work that I do with people. She ordered my first book right there on her phone and even booked a private session.

Sarah's genuine warmth and nurturing energy lights up a room. People instantly feel better around her. For the more sensitive and intuitive though, it's palpable that she is wrestling with something internally that deeply troubles her. About six weeks later, we had our first remote video session.

"Hi, Sarah. Nice to see you again."

"Likewise. Can I ask you something that I've been dying to know?"

"Sure.

"How are you able to do what you do?"

"It's how I choose to be of service."

"I mean not give up on people?"

This question, like everything we give birth to, simply reveals our inner life. Like showing your hand when playing cards.

"I don't have any expectations."

"How is that possible?"

"Accept yourself fully, now, and you will tangibly realize you are whole and complete, always. Expectations will literally cease to exist."

Timeless truths run counter to low-frequency programming. The subconscious, patterned, egoic mind is resistance to "what is." Upon nonacceptance of the Real You—the only truth—the subconscious, patterned mind immediately reacts by running its programs, thus creating mental/emotional/physical distress.

Sarah sighed. "I can't. I've tried. It doesn't work. I've been mistreated my entire life. How can I feel good about myself? Everyone is always trying to take advantage of me, and I don't know how to say no."

Sarah's mental and emotional dam finally broke. After decades of feeling worn down by others, her deep sadness, hurt, and betrayal spilled out. I remained fully present and opened my heart to provide a high-frequency space for her as she sobbed.

"It's okay. It's okay."

After a moment or two, Sarah began to regain control. The victimhood identity produced by the patterned, subconscious, egoic mind doesn't allow for anything other than a momentary reprieve.

She wiped the tears away from her cheeks and eyes. "I'm so embarrassed. I can't believe I'm acting like this in front of you."

"No worries," I said. "I get a lot more crying than I do applause."

We both laughed.

I tapped my chin with a wry grin. "Maybe I should find a new line of work."

The laughter settled Sarah down, and she continued.

"I don't want to be this way anymore. I feel like I can't control how I react no matter how hard I try. I just give in all the time. I feel totally defeated."

"I understand."

"RJ, I do meditation and yoga. I understand about energy and ascension. Why can't I do this?"

"You can; you just haven't been taught properly, that's all. It's very simple to do, and the results are tangible, lasting, and profound."

Sarah was eager to hear more, so I continued, "We cannot transcend what we do not see or understand. The subconscious mind is what cocreates our reality—far more than our conscious thoughts. That is because we only think/emote and do in relation to our subconscious programming and egoic mind. The deep-rooted subconscious mind involves 'imprinting' upon our lower astral body. The astral body is where very deep-rooted indentations and identifications reside. Think of the astral body like a higher-frequency radio station than our mental, emotional, etheric, and physical bodies receive transmissions on. Whatever information gets imprinted upon and within our astral then trickles down the stairs like an energetic slinky and informs and feeds the lower-frequency bands or radio stations that are the mental, emotional, etheric, and physical bodies. Hence, you have no conscious control over yourself."

"Is this why it feels like I can't say no or control myself?"

"Yes, some of this imprinting is consciously done by your misidentification with them, like a belief or experience. That imprinting becomes part of your EMI limitation program, which runs every time you have a thought. Some imprints or indentations are big enough boulders upon your energetic bedspread that conscious misidentification with them is not required for it to affect you. Because it has become embedded within your body of energy, it becomes part of your subconscious, patterned mind."

"This is mind-boggling. Can you teach me how to overcome this?"

"I can but your transcendence will be solely dependent upon your courage, open-mindedness, and dedication to the teachings."

"I need to do this. I'm all in."

The very next day, I saw an email from Sarah not even twenty-four hours since our session. The subject line of the email was just one word: *WOW*. Here is what she shared with me:

"RJ, I can't believe what I have realized about myself after doing the notebook exercise for just one day! Everything I do is because of my subconscious, patterned mind and EMI. Everything! This has been completely eye-opening. I feel so different. Like I'm floating. This is incredible! My sadness and hurt are disappearing.

Here's what I wrote in my notebook."

FEELING UPSET AFTER GETTING OFF THE PHONE WITH MY MOM.

Question: Why do I feel upset?

Answer: Because my mom doesn't understand me, ever.

Question: Why do I care that my mom doesn't understand me?

Answer: Because she's supposed to be there for me.

Question: Why do I care if my mom isn't there for me?

Answer: Because it makes me feel like I am alone and lost.

Question: Why am I afraid to be alone?

Answer: Because it's too scary.

Question: Why do I feel it's too scary?

Answer: Because I don't want to see myself.

Questions: Why do I not want to see myself?

Answer: Because I know am capable of so much more than this.

"This shifted my mind. I could feel something opening inside me, expanding. I kept going..."

Question: Why do I choose to hold myself back?

Answer: Because it's easier to blame others and focus on them.

Question: Why do I think this way?

Answer: So I don't have to be responsible for my life. It's easier to be disappointed in and blame others for my life than to be fearless and strong.

Question: Why am I afraid to be fearless?

Answer: So I don't have to face failure. Not having success in my life is not my fault if I keep focused on validation and pleasing others. That's why I'm depressed. I always look outside myself so that I don't have to focus on me and finally take control and responsibility for my life.

Sarah continued in her email, "RJ, I have felt depressed and lived like a victim my whole life. I did it because I was programmed to seek approval, guidance, help, validation, and permission from everyone, especially my mom. I see it now. I never needed it. And the deep sadness, the heaviness, is leaving me, finally.

"I am going to be Wonder Woman by the time I am done with the notebook exercise, lol. Thank you so much! You have changed my life in just one day!!!"

By bringing her subconscious, patterned, egoic mind into her conscious view, Sarah changed her life in one day! She is no longer conditioned to disempower herself repeatedly. She has finally given herself permission—freedom—to live her life on her terms.

Summary

With this new and deeper understanding about how the subconscious mind dictates your every behavior, as well as how to bring that deep invisible programming into your conscious awareness, your life is now your own! No more reacting with predictive limiting responses to situations. No more recycling experiences with the same unsatisfying results in your personal growth, intimate relationships, or business endeavors.

This can be done by simply questioning your:

- Thoughts (Why do I think that?)
- Emotions (Why do I feel that way?)

- Actions (Why am I doing this?)
- Behaviors (Why am I continually operating in this way?)

Until you uncover the core motivation driving each notion, you will only repeat them. Through the simple yet powerful notebook exercise, you break the spell your patterned, subconscious mind has over you. You have finally unmasked the shadow puppeteer that's been pulling your strings. You have the ability and protocols to easily illuminate and disempower your subconscious, patterned, egoic mind. Now, nothing can hold you back. Your infinite potential, inner peace, limitless capacity to create, love, and enjoy your life has been taken back by its rightful owner: you!

In the next chapter, you are going to discover the universal habits of subconscious programming and egoic identifications.

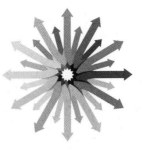

Chapter 4

Signs You Are Dissolving Your Subconscious Programming

There are many tangible indicators that you are regaining dominion over your subconscious, patterned, egoic mind. In essence, this process is like letting go of all the baggage and knickknacks you acquired from a very long, strange trip! By doing so, you are finally returning home, and from a metaphysical perspective, that is exactly what is happening. Your direct return to conscious mind/body attunement to the Immortal Self will illuminate a myriad of mental, emotional, and physical imbalances, habits, and patterns that do not belong to you.

This shedding of temporarily acquired baggage and tchotchkes is crucial to the process of realignment with what you really are: the Self. Along with your understanding of the subsequent observations, what we are about to go over in detail is all part of your long journey home. Knowing what many of these universal and needed changes look and feel like will help keep you from falling back into patterned, subconscious programming and egoic identifications.

The only constant is change, and yet you remain. Do not fear it. It is necessary for the data points (experiences/relationships/events) in your life plan to have the space to manifest. Your nonattachment to whatever pops up onto the screen of your consciousness allows the flow of existence to work in total alignment with your highest good.

It is your resistance (programming) that prevents "what is." Remember, resistance is not germane to the sacred geometric building blocks of "what is." You mistakenly create resistance, and that is what causes you to suffer. Do not resist your own life plan, your own flowering, by fearing and avoiding change. You will miss the tangible beauty, endless perfection, and total fullness inherent within every single moment.

Here are the top twenty-five signs you are deprogramming your subconscious, patterned, egoic mind:

#1: You Desire Alone Time

Desiring alone time is a healthy inclination to maintain energetic hygiene. Most of us don't even remember what alone time is. That's because we have replaced any natural proclivities toward Self-care with programmed low-frequency habits. Alone time is not binge-watching TV, scrolling social media, nonstop text messaging, or incessant online research. None of that is alone time nor is it rejuvenating.

Wanting to stop taking in a constant stream of free radicals (information) and ceasing to commingle your energies with others is a sign the Self is becoming a tangible presence in your life. Remember, the Self is whole and complete as it is. It simply desires to marinate within its own essence.

Do not fear or work against the desire to be alone. It's an indicator of Self-awareness, mature independence, intuitive wisdom, and nonattachment. These are all fragrances of the divine nectar emanating from your heart. Embrace them.

#2: You Feel Like You Have Less in Common with Other People

Welcome to the club! On a much deeper level, what is happening when you feel like you have less in common with people is that your outer human personality—the subconscious, patterned, egoic mind, which is the currency of this world—is losing its control over you.

As you shed your programming, the previously shared commiserations, identifications, and interests that were the common ground between you and others dissipate. You no longer feel the low-frequency connection you once shared with others.

On a significantly deeper level, your clarity, calmness, connectivity, and communion with authenticity is being turned back on. In essence, you are getting closer to everything and everyone at the core of their being. They may not be operating this way, so they may very well feel a disconnection from you as well.

If I asked you to touch one of my newly charged crystals (I love charging crystals) and tell me what it tangibly feels like and what physical qualities you can perceive, your assessment and feedback would be wholly inaccurate if you were wearing three pairs of mittens while you did it. By deprogramming your subconscious, egoic mind, you are removing your mittens. You know yourself and everything else you encounter more accurately and authentically.

Now with your mittens discarded, the experience of both yourself and the crystal is totally different. That's what it's like when you do this work. You are removing your subconscious and egoic filters. Those who are not taking off their multiple mittens don't feel the same to you, and you don't feel the same to them either. This explains why you will feel like you have less in common with people and vice versa. Check the boxes on a mitten and crystal analogies all in one go!

#3: Your Hobbies and Interests Change

What has been dictating and driving your behavior up until now—subconscious indentations and egoic identifications—has probably gone uninvestigated and unchecked for many years, maybe decades. This is an aspect of not evolving your consciousness with the greatest efficacy. Once a habitual limiting pattern has infected any area of your life, it will eventually infect other facets of your life as well, even hobbies and interests.

Your leanings and predilections will most likely change because your mittens are off and your newfound tangible Self-awareness and greater Self-control over your mind/body complex will lead you in new directions. You may still have an interest in previous hobbies, but your experience when participating in them may very well be different.

I have found that many people start to become interested in higher consciousness metaphysics as well as being of service. Some are inexplicably drawn to creative endeavors. Simply be aware of your changing landscape as it pertains to hobbies and interests. Be open and allow whatever it is you feel passionate about. Do not lament over what no longer holds interest for you—be it a person, place, or thing.

#4: You Cherish Simple Pleasures Much More than Before

You may find the need to satiate previous mental, emotional, and physical programming begin to leave you. It is often replaced with the direct, tangible, and simple pleasures of life. That is because, like Indiana Jones on a quest to unearth a lost, ancient, and sacred treasure, you are discovering what has always been hidden inside you: clarity, peace, completeness, and the towering immortal presence of eternal divinity.

You may no longer feel the previously never-ending energetic toll of incessantly needing to be productive. Stimulation, be it pain/pleasure or even the adrenaline rush that your subconscious mind and egoic identity endlessly requires, no longer holds sway over you. That's because the Real You is freedom itself and seeks nothing but the tangible recognition of its own fully illuminated presence.

Now that the indentations and identifications within your energetic bedspread no longer need your energy, you may very well take great joy in the simplicity of pure being—being with yourself or with nature, watching animals play, sharing a meal, reading a good book, or experiencing a hearty laugh. Inherent in simplicity is an elegance, grace, and power, and that is the Real You, my friends, to the core.

#5: You Are Less Negative and Not as Adversely Affected by the World

Your subconscious indentations and egoic identifications are the tangible experience of low-frequency programming and illusion. World culture (what passes for it due to massive perception management) is built from and upon this misprogramming. It is why the driving force behind your daily behavior feels so utterly unsatisfying and pointless to the Real You.

With all perceivable phenomena no longer misidentified as the Self, you become less affected by what awareness is aware of. The indentations and identifications are no longer weighing on you. Subsequently, your inclination is no longer negativity or low-frequency oriented.

You are now operating above and beyond your patterned, subconscious, egoic mind. Therefore, you are less affected by what you perceive. What used to trigger and rock you to the core now only registers as passing phenomena. Feeling more grounded within your authenticity—not triggered by subconscious programming—is why this change is occurring.

#6: You No Longer See Anyone or Anything in the Same Way as Before

Your subconscious programming and EMI are layers upon layers of misperception, misunderstanding, and misidentification. In this state, it is impossible to have the tangible, direct experience of the Self. Therefore, it is impossible to tangibly experience anything as it is either. How can we understand anything if we do not understand the Self? It is what gives birth to all.

As the mittens of subconscious programming and egoic identifications are taken off, your inner experience of Self—and therefore reality—changes. As the Self deepens, you concurrently and synergistically will experience the outside world through different eyes. Think of it this way: you can change one hundred times in a single day and still be wearing the same clothes.

Embrace your new level of Self-awareness but refrain from the habit of judgment. That Self-destructive programmed habit only drops your own frequency. Accept your new state of being with grace, humility, and courage. Anything less would be a return to subconscious programming and egoic behaviors.

#7: You No Longer Believe/Disbelieve in What You Are Told to Believe/Disbelieve

As the subconscious (energetic bedspread) is freed from indentations and the EMI from identifications, something truly amazing begins to happen: clarity. Your intuitive knowingness now has a greater and more accurate say in "what is." The subconscious, patterned, egoic mind is but a petulant child beside the towering presence of timeless wisdom.

The most beautiful thing in the world is to own your own mind. This is liberation. You will no longer be under the spell of coercion, manipulation, greed, and fear. Believing is seeing, not the other way around.

The truth does not require your participation. Lies do. As you continue with your coursework as outlined in this book, your programmed inclination to believe, obey, and conform will leave you. You will be connected to something infinitely deeper and far more powerful than societal pressures. It's called the Real You.

#8: You Feel the Desire to Wake Up Others

We all possess a natural inclination to assist. It is woven within the very fabric of our being to share. That's because, metaphysically speaking, at the deepest level, we truly are one consciousness. That is why everything is designed for us to come together. If you find yourself feeling the desire to assist others in waking up, it's because you are waking up.

Let's look at the desire to help wake others from a different perspective. Whatever someone is going through, they are experiencing it because they need to have that experience. Otherwise, they would not be having the experience. There is something that Soul needs to learn, and that is why that experience is occurring. You may not need to learn that lesson, but someone else does for their spiritual growth. Just be there for them so they can move through it in their own way and in their own time.

Remember, if you feel the desire to fix someone or something, that is because you are viewing life as broken. Nothing is broken. That Soul has not failed. It is simply experiencing delayed success. The way in which they have or are currently operating has brought them to a particular juncture. From a human perspective, you may label this person or situation as broken, but I assure you that is only on the surface. Nothing is broken because life does not need fixing. Both helping and fixing come from a subconscious, patterned, egoic perspective.

To serve flows directly to the Self. When you serve, you see life as whole and complete. Feel the tangible difference in energetic qualities of helping/fixing and when you serve. Being in service is sharing, and it feels completely different. It comes from an unending source: the Real You. Helping and fixing is exhausting due to its subconscious, egoic origins, while serving is uplifting and energizing. Never forget the difference between helping, fixing, and serving.

#9: You Lose Interest in Partying, Group Gatherings, and Gossip

The currency of humanity is the low-frequency, programmed mind. As you deprogram yourself, you will naturally rise in frequency. The allure of intermingling with groups that possess a party mindset or gossiping is extremely low frequency. Losing the desire to engage in these activities is a healthy sign and nothing to lament over. It indicates a deeper and more direct connection with the complete Self. This portends further expansion of your higher mind.

Being freed from the desires that were part of your patterned subconscious and your egoic mind should not be met with resistance. Embrace and allow your new moment-to-moment state of being. You are no longer the same conditioned individual you were before. Some desires, like the previously mentioned, will simply leave you or, at the very least, will have little sway over you. Notice the tangible difference between how you feel now in comparison to the old desire to engage in those behaviors.

There is no need to give in to peer pressure or revert to old habits. There is also no need to shun something automatically. Be honest with yourself. As certain desires leave you, know that they have left because they no longer serve you. Do not reach or grasp for what is not present within you.

#10: Your Circle of Friends Gets Smaller

As you deprogram the patterned mind, your vibration changes. You will no longer be on the same frequency that you—and most of your friends—were previously on. Oddly enough, as you become more expansive and freer internally, your circle of friends will shrink. That is because the common ground has shifted. You are no longer on the same dance floor, exhibiting the same old moves. You now hear a different song than your previous dance partners currently do. You may even discover you are at a completely different venue. That was a festival of analogies!

If your circle of friends gets smaller or morphs, simply embrace and accept it. Do not create resistance toward "what is" as this will cause you and others suffering. Deprogramming your subconscious, patterned, egoic mind is an individual endeavor. In the beginning it can feel lonely, especially as the circle of friends shrinks. This reduction in your outer circle is being replaced with the greater gnosis

(Self-knowledge) and authenticity. Soon enough you will discover other travelers on the very same journey.

#11: You No Longer Label Yourself by Indentations or Identifications

You may find that how you saw yourself prior to working with the teachings and understandings in this book has shifted. That's because what is now driving your behavior is a more direct expression of the Self. The Self (from a metaphysical perspective) has no personalized identity. It also has no name, form, or image. The Self has qualities, attributes, and talents, which we will get into later, but not an identity to label.

As the marbles, rocks, and boulders are removed from your energetic bedspread, you will think, act, feel, and behave differently. Victimhood, for example, will finally be seen for what it is: a concept born of the unawakened mind. You didn't come from here and you certainly didn't come to stay, so there is no point in trying to fit. There is nothing here that is authentically you, including all indentations and identifications we call labels.

Experiencing yourself as formless, free, and unconditioned is "what is." Your Self-talk creates your reality. Be extremely mindful of what you say to yourself. Words are precious, but what is even more precious is the silence underneath them. Listen to the voice inside that doesn't use words to speak and the mysteries of existence will reveal themselves.

#12: You Become More Intuitive

The subconscious, patterned, egoic mind is a looped program of indentations and identifications. As you remove/repair/transcend the indentations and identifications, your mind is no longer locked in repeat. Your energy is no longer being consumed by your previous predictive programming.

The patterned subconscious prevents the aroma (attributes and talents) of the Self from wafting its fragrance of intuitive know-ingness into your awareness. That's because your programmed mind is not receptive to what is. Higher intuitive functions, such as clairsentience, clairvoyance, and claircognizance, can come online as you deprogram. That's because your unconditioned awareness is expanding.

It is important to listen and foster your growing sense of intu-ition. Intuition is an act of listening. Pay attention. It can be subtle, but as the mind becomes less preoccupied with thought and the body with sensations, your intuition will become tangible. Do not seek confirmation, approval, or validation from others. Intuition is learning to trust your Self. The Self is your knowingness, your intu-ition, and your higher intuitive functions. It's all the Real You.

#13: You Become Calmer and More Introspective

As you remove indentations and identifications through the teach-ings of this book, you regain dominion over the mind/body com-plex as well as your body of energy. This greater command over your Total Self (sentience + energy) naturally results in being calmer and more introspective. You are now walking and living a true spiritual path. Spiritual growth is the point of being here, period.

Our natural state is to be peaceful, wise, and fully present. That equates to total mental clarity and complete emotional stability. Our natural state—what is, sans any electromagnetic interference or EMI—promotes Self-knowledge. Becoming comfortable with being calm and introspective is a tangible sign that you are deprogram-ming your subconscious, patterned, egoic mind. Fall in love with the depth and serenity of the Self.

Allow the seedlings of Self-introspection to take root. Now that you have more of your energy at your conscious disposal, use it to be creative. Journaling is a great way to further unearth the sacred trea-sures within you that have been covered by earthly indentations and identifications.

#14: Everything You Thought You Knew —Believed In—Is No Longer True

As your patterned, subconscious, egoic mind, which blindfolds your awareness and imprisons your love, regains its pristine state, the beliefs that slithered their way into your mind start to lose their fangs. The hissing voice wrapped around your consciousness, seducing you into submission and conformity—or suffer the viper's sting of societal rejection and egoic condemnation—has lost its poisonous venom.

What supports and reinforces the patterned subconscious and the egoic mind are your justifications for them. As you remove them from your energetic bedspread, you will no longer believe in their authenticity, and therefore, they will hold no gravitas. What once was ingrained and shrouded in darkness is now revealed by the clarity of introspection, intuitive awareness, and non-identification.

As the patterned, subconscious mind is brought into conscious awareness, your beliefs and, subsequently, your thoughts will change. What was driving your behavior has been removed. Blind belief and egoic identifications are like a dirty windshield. Take the time to adjust to seeing the path ahead through a very different lens. That counts as another analogy for those of you keeping score.

#15: Career Interests May Change

The Self contains the talents and abilities—as well as the life plan—within it. It is totally normal for your interests to morph, and that could include a possible career change. Do not run, avoid, or chase changes. They are part of your awakening and expansion. Embrace them courageously and with an open mind. Change happens so you can see your unfolding life plan.

Changes in a career can often cause stress. That's because evolution is not part of the predictive programming. Therefore, it is automatically eschewed and feared. The programmed mind only accepts and works with its indentations and identifications. Both the EMI and the subconscious, patterned mind fear and reject anything out-side of their respective limitations (comfort zone).

Do not be surprised if your career interests lean toward being of service in one form or another. Many people I have shared the note-book exercise with find themselves compelled to assist others. That is because they have freed themselves, and it often follows that they want the same for all.

#16: Your Connection and Affinity for Nature Increases

Working with nature is a directive woven within the core of your essence. Embrace it. It's your patterned, subconscious, egoic mind that has diverted your direct and tangible connection from this. Nature calling you is a great indicator that your energetic bedspread is returning to its original purity and, along with it, so is your capac-ity to love and serve.

Because you are getting in touch with your true nature directly, you may very well be drawn to other direct forms of authenticity as well. If you are drawn to walk on the grass barefoot or go for a hike (wear shoes on the hike, please!), follow your impulse. Watching or playing with animals, relaxing at the beach, or paddling out on a boat to take in the serene surroundings are all healing and rejuvenat-ing on the deepest levels.

Examine what it is that pulls you toward reconnecting with nature. Discover where within you this impulse arises. Make it a goal to tan-gibly understand this pull as it relates to your direct being-ness. What you are discovering about the nature of the Self is infinitely more valu-able, precious, and beyond what any book learning can ever give you.

#17: Intimate Personal Relationships May End or Evolve

As you remove and repair the indentations and identifications within your body of energy and patterned, egoic mind, your sense of Self radically changes. Just like how removing pairs of mittens from your hands lets you experience objects differently, you now experience yourself differently. You will subsequently experience everyone and everything differently as well. Nowhere will this be more obvious and apparent than the dynamic between you and those very close to you.

As you awaken to greater authenticity and Self-awareness and ascend the frequencies, you must acknowledge and accept the end of all relationships not founded on authenticity. This can mean letting go of a long-standing partnership. It can also mean the ending of your previous dynamic and the birth of a new one between you and your significant other.

Either way, embrace "what is." Long-standing friendships can and will change as you change. The deepest connections are those built upon loyalty, friendship, respect, and trust. Platonic relationships whose foundations are built upon the granite of truth, loyalty, and friendship will never crack. Intimate relationships that have those embedded within the fabric of their union will withstand the sea of change. In fact, they will become stronger, deeper, and more fulfilling because of it.

#18: You Seek Inner Tangible Truth Rather than the Opinions of Belief

The idea of deprogramming your subconscious, patterned, egoic mind for the unawakened immediately invokes fear for what they will lose. I am sorry to say their fear is well founded. There will be great loss. Loss of anxiety, depression, neediness, unworthiness, limited intuition, impulsivity, short temperedness, fear, greed, anger, abandonment issues, reactionary outbursts, unhealthy habits, repetitive and undesirable outcomes, negative Self-talk, and the recycling of unsavory experiences. If you fear the loss of those things, then put this book down.

Your own BS will no longer be palatable, even to you. And when I say *BS*, I mean belief systems. The tangible recognition of what rings true at your core will be your new guidepost. The high and low tides within the shifting sea of illusions and beliefs will no longer ensnare you in their currents. You are now anchored in truth. The Self is the only reality and the indomitable lighthouse that never goes dark. You are now the one person everyone can count on, starting with yourself.

Own your own mind. This is life's greatest treasure and beauty. As your programmed behavior and reactionary state of being begins to leave you, realize that truth has never been out of your grasp. You were simply used to reaching out rather than tangibly realizing you are already it.

#19: You Desire Better Mental and Emotional Health

One of the incredible and lasting benefits of doing transformative inner work is the ability to quickly and more accurately recognize where there is room for growth. Wanting to experience greater mental clarity and emotional stability is the hallmark of an awakening mind. Desiring far greater facility to be present and calm is the Self making its immortal and invincible presence known.

The Self is meditation. The patterned, subconscious, egoic mind is the opposite. It can't stop craving, even for peace, just to get a respite from itself. The patterned mind is the tangible experience of no Self-control. It even "performs meditation," but it's done as a task whose box can now be checked off as a quantifiable metric under the guise of productivity. That way, it can justifiably return to its perpetual trancelike hunger state. The statements "I am meditating" and "I am not meditating" both reinforce the illusion of the EMI.

Better mental and emotional health will often lead to enhanced physical health. If the desire is true and coming from an authentic place within you, it will start at the core of your being and infuse your mind. At that point, you will bathe the impulse with e-motion (energy in motion). Then, and only then, will the body be sufficiently charged to act.

#20: You Are More Protective of Your Energy

Because you are now acutely aware of how your energetic bedspread has been impacted, you will naturally be mindful of its well-being. Because of the work you're doing with this book, this understanding has now become part of your conscious awareness. You are now far more Self-aware and that includes awareness of your more subtle body of energy, not just your physical vehicle.

What is interesting is that tangible Self-awareness automatically leads to greater awareness of the Total You (sentience + energy). You do not have to do anything outside of deprogramming the subconscious, patterned, egoic mind for this realization. Being more aware and mindful of your subtle energies is an ancillary effect of the profound, effective, and expansive inner work you are currently doing.

In part 3, you are going to discover a revolutionary energy diagnostic system. You will learn how to quantifiably measure the effects of stimulus upon you as well as learn a reliable system to help manage your energy bank account. This will give you a simple, robust, actionable, effective, and repeatable process to keep you in alignment, true to yourself, and acutely aware of your energy.

#21: You Value Yourself and Others Far More

This will be quite a switch from valuing the brainwashing, misidentifications, and bodily behaviors of the patterned, subconscious mind. This may very well be the first time you begin to experience the Real You. Welcome home. By eschewing the limiting habit of getting stuck in time by creating a past or a future through incessant thought, you will begin to hold yourself in significantly higher regard.

As you cease to quantify your day by how much of your subconscious programming you obeyed and temporarily satiated, you now sense at the deepest levels that you are already whole and complete. Your innate being-ness—the I AM—is this highest value. You are it, and from there, everything flows. Once this becomes tangible, you will also realize this innate I AM is not only the highest value, but it is also universal with all existence. This eternal truth will translate into allowance and compassion for all life. The Master within is now rising!

The value inherent in greater Self-awareness is the spaciousness and acceptance you will now have for yourself and others. The value you feel inside will never again be transferred to humanistic misperceptions, misunderstanding, and misidentifications. It cannot be hijacked or conferred onto something or someone. It is you and you are it, always. And all "life" is an expression of that very same I AM that birthed you.

#22: You Don't Crave Constant Stimulation and Distractions

Your desire to distract yourself endlessly is to escape the tyranny of your subconscious, patterned, egoic mind. You distract yourself because the way in which you are operating is unbearable to the Real You. Distractions, for many of us, are the only way to distance ourselves from the misery and deeply unsatisfying nature of our programmed and limited body-consciousness state of being. Not anymore.

Craving distraction is simply your grooves, indentations, and identifications needing energy that you refuse to give. Remember, without attention (and attention is energy) things die. Real meditation eventually destroys all imbalances because those imbalances never get fed any attention/energy. There is a reason every authentic Master advocates fasting and meditation—it purifies mind/body/spirit.

The day you fall in love with your own inner stillness and silence is the day you no longer live in bondage. Your life will finally be your own. No more craving constant stimulation or distractions. Everything that is in vibrational alignment with your Self will be drawn unto you. There will never be a need for stimulation or distraction.

#23: You Are Less Scared by So-Called Failure

What we call failure is simply delayed success. When you no longer fear failure or success, you are free to create without the limitation of expectation. By liberating yourself from the subconscious, patterned, egoic mind, limitless imagination is tangibly known once more. This is the true nature of "what is," and you are a complete fractal of this limitlessness. Similarly, like a hologram, the fractal contains the totality.

When more of your body of energy and mind are commandeered by their rightful owner—the Real You—fear in all its forms gets alchemized. That's because there is nothing for an immortal and perfect creator being to fear. The poisonous beliefs of fear must be planted, nurtured, and reinforced. Without it, as you are realizing, your true nature begins to take hold. Freedom!

Feeling empowered to live your life authentically is a tangible side effect of greater Self-awareness and so is not worrying about an outcome. The fullness of the Self is available within every single moment of your existence. Trust and faith will replace fear and doubt as you continue to disarm the subconscious, patterned, egoic mind into complete subservience and submission.

#24: You Are Determined
and Not Deterred or Defeated

Determination allows you to tangibly experience your will. Harnessing it is your will power. Feeling determined is the residue of greater clarity and focus. It is a natural byproduct of having more dominion over your body/mind/energy complex. Let your newfound determination carry you across previously feared and unchartered waters.

The subconscious, patterned, egoic mind can only operate within very narrow bandwidths. It keeps you subservient, submissive, and subhuman. Your own patterned mind keeps you in line—literally and figuratively. As your energetic bedspread returns to its naturally robust and unencumbered state, you will feel less deterred and more

determined. The decreasing "weight" of your indentations and identifications is why and just cause for sincere gratitude.

Do not withhold your immense power from your limitless nature.
Humanity does not consciously remember the enlightened civilizations we created for ourselves. It is your ancient future once again.
Your determination—your will—being directed by your true nature
will yield inner fulfillment and deep purpose. Be the joyous witness to
the depth of your own majesty and divine power.

#25: Your Most Fervent Desire Is for Peace and Happiness

As you shed the programming of the subconscious, patterned, egoic
mind, all the trauma, fears, and desires that were never yours to
begin with leave you. None of it will seem authentic anymore. That
is because the human character who was transfixed by the programming wasn't authentically you either. The unease and discomfort of
being perpetually misprogrammed has been lifted. And with it, a
great discovery is made.

Pure being-ness—the Self—is eternal peace, equanimity, and
happiness. There is no effort required to be what you already are. A
bird doesn't have to try to be a bird, it's a bird. You do not have to try
to be yourself, you are yourself. All your effort is in being something
that you are not: your subconscious, patterned, egoic identity.

Accept the Real You fully, and you will effortlessly be present.
Inner peace and ever-present happiness will become tangibly known
and normalized because it's you—without effort, straining, or trying. Surrender to the truth. Your highest desire and achievement are
already within you.

Summary

The signs that you are deprogramming your subconscious, patterned, egoic mind will be all around you. They will present themselves within your moment-to-moment existence. What you do, how

you do it, and even the "who" that is performing the actions will feel different. Your actual thought process will change because thoughts are always in relation to indentations and identifications. As you deprogram, those free radicals are removed, and subsequently your thought patterns change. Deprogramming your subconscious, egoic mind changes your brain waves and therefore, how you experience and create your life.

Prior to deprogramming, you may have relied upon outside sources in myriad ways. Now that you have reclaimed your own mind, the process in which you create your life could be very different. Self-confidence, independence, intuition, and inner resolve may be far more tangible. No need to reach for something or someone when you now know you already and always have everything you need.

Synchronicity, which in the past you may have labeled as luck (good or bad), coincidence, or happenstance due to your subconscious programming, will be more and more obvious. The grand plan, your grand plan, is unfolding right before your eyes. It's tangibly more and more obvious now because you have removed your blinders, namely your programmed mind. The screen of your consciousness has been cleaned. Clarity and connectivity can no longer be denied, written off, or ignored. This is proof that you have deprogrammed your subconscious mind.

Feeling more in flow with yourself and not in fear, resistance, or doubt about life—your life—is a powerful sign of deprogramming. Things coming together mentally, emotionally, and physically is proof that your blockages—your programmed mind—have been deleted. When this starts to occur, your outer life and parts of it, such as business, love, and friendships, will require less and less effort. That is because the one who was always straining and efforting—your ego/mind/identity, which is caused by electro/magnetic/interference—is less real and present in your life. The static is gone. This is confirmation that you have deprogrammed your subconscious, patterned, egoic mind.

Part 2

Becoming the Real You

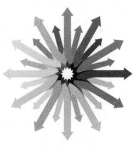

Chapter 5
How to Express the Real You 24–7

I get asked all the time: How am I supposed to live my life? What are the guidelines? What is truly the best way to live? In other words: What am I supposed to do and why? Let's look at how we can immediately and impactfully address this.[5]

Being and expressing the Real You is certainly not possible through the indentations and identifications of low-frequency conditioning. The best way to live is very simple: do what you tangibly know to be true and expect no results. This is the single most important understanding in terms of being able to express and be the Real You—always.

When we speak about truth being tangible, there is a felt energetic quality to truth. There is a knowingness deep within your heart, where your sentience—what you really are—resides within your body. This knowingness is the exact opposite of mental and emotional conditioning, both of which have their origination everywhere but within you. That's the difference between knowing and conditioning.

....
5. This chapter was taken from a lecture/presentation I performed live for my students July 14, 2022.

Your true character, your morality, and your ethics, you come into this life with them. They are part of your essence. This is what I'm referring to in terms of tangibly knowing to be true within you. Live in alignment with this and have no expectations from the action. By operating properly (perpetual presence/flow state), you remain free from a past and future and therefore not bound by the limitations of time.

Do What You Tangibly Know to Be True and Expect No Results

Let's explore the depth and meaning of this statement further. The above statement allows you to stay in the present moment—perpetually—because you don't have an expectation of any future results, nor are you burdened by ruminations of the past. This is moment-to-moment, pure being-ness. You then simply take your being-ness and put it into your doing-ness. This is the flow state. Do what you tangibly know to be true within this moment, and then the next moment, and then the next moment, and then the next moment, etc.

Thinking, which is the movement of the past projected forward into what you call the future, traps you in "time," which does not authentically exist. Both the concepts of past and of future only exist within your subconscious, patterned, egoic mind, which is the cause of your suffering.

This higher-frequency way of living keeps you in the act of perpetual presence and creativity, which is how an awakened immortal creator being plays optimally. Stay within this pure presence, perpetual being-ness, and perpetual creativity, flowing from moment to moment, by tangibly doing what you know to be true without expecting any results.

Being-ness and Doing-ness

By taking your being-ness and putting it into your doing-ness, you are truly expressing the Real You. When you live this way, you are free from conditioning because you are no longer addicted to creating the delusions of a past or future. This is how to best operate all the time, 24–7, in every situation: personal, business, family, friends, and inner dialogue. Results, in and of themselves, are inconsequential and always based upon a past and future. The process of being masterful with yourself is the ultimate achievement, not any result from it.

This is how to live authentically in a low-frequency, inauthentic world: doing what you tangibly know to be true, not living by what you have been conditioned to believe, think, and obey. This is how to transcend the limitations of your conditioning.

Work with that one truth and you shall remain eternally free. Live this way with everyone, always. Do what you tangibly know to be true, and only speak about what you tangibly know to be true. This is the ultimate because you are now operating at your truest and highest level. Your subconscious, patterned, egoic mind (suffering) will no longer dictate your life.

The Fragmentation and Compartmentalization of the Self

Most of us experience ourselves and therefore life from a fragmented, disjointed, and compartmentalized viewpoint. Look at how you act, behave, and speak in a business setting, for example. Then look at how you act, behave, and speak with a family member. And then the same thing in terms of maybe with your children. And then how you act and behave with your friends. How about with your mom and dad? What about your inner dialogue and the way in which you behave toward yourself?

When you start to look at this, you realize it's impossible to be true to yourself if you behave and operate a certain way within one fragmentation, behave and operate in another way within a different fragmentation, and so on and so on.

Think about your Self-talk; think about the nature of the dynamic between your partner or your kids or your friends, relatives, neighbors, business partners, etc. How many different characters are you playing? And how many of those are directly and authentically you?

It is impossible to be the Real You because those characters/roles have hijacked your mind and body. Are you ever being truthful, or are you constantly trying to squeeze yourself into some compart-mentalization and fragmentation of conditioning? Is everything you endeavor done to meet some sort of programmed ideal for happi-ness and/or security? Is it all a feckless attempt to satiate your per-petually ravenous subconscious, patterned, egoic mind?

Let's look at these life situations. Are you incessantly trying to navigate and control your life and every situation? Do you manipu-late others with your energy so they agree, comply, or see things the way you do? Remember, if you try to control and manipulate others with your energy, it's because you have been manipulated and con-trolled by your programming.

Programmed to Control Out of Fear and Greed

If you're trying to control a situation, it's because you are controlled. And if you are controlled through beliefs, through your indenta-tions and identifications, that's not the Real You. In fact, it's quite the opposite.

When you cease trying to try to control your life, situations, and others, you have stepped into being and expressing the Real You. You're no longer interested in a specific outcome, whether it's per-sonal, business, or even with yourself, your family, or your kids, believe it or not. That's because you are already at peace, feel ful-filled, and are grateful for now. Now you are enjoying life because the sense of play has returned.

Stop trying to control others to see if they fit into your life. If you truly want to see somebody, I mean really get to know them, simply let them do whatever they want, whenever they want. Only then will you finally see them for who they are. It's just like when you shake a snow globe and can't see inside it very well; your clarity regarding others only occurs when you cease to stir them. Do the same with yourself.

Due to your inner fragmentation, separation, and compartmentalization, you end up behaving a certain way in certain situations. Only when you stop doing any of that will you finally feel like yourself. Only then will you be experiencing and expressing the Real You.

Without realizing it, you have become a puppet to various puppeteers. If you drop your personal agenda in every one of these different fragmented realities that you create for yourself, what is it that remains? What is it that would then be fully present in every one of these circumstances within your life? The Real You. Character, clarity, confidence, calmness, connectivity, courage, and communion will be tangibly known once again.

Being and Expressing the Real You Is the Only Achievement

You are programmed to believe that through some sort of achievement, becoming, or recognition (often justified by any means necessary), happiness/security will finally be yours. When really the thing that you're trying to get out of the experience is what you already and eternally are before you endeavor to do anything, which is the experience of the immortal and divine Real You.

Your happiness, lasting peace, and completeness exist before and only without the compartmentalization, fragmentation, and separation of the patterned, subconscious, egoic mind. With all the beliefs, concepts, and roles you play with your parents, partner, kids, friends, siblings, business associates, neighbors, etc., there is no way to truly be happy, peaceful, and content while being that internally divided. It's impossible.

In fact, you are constantly torturing yourself—and probably others—through the incessant and addictive manipulation and coercion of yourself—and therefore others—to get some sort of result that you're programmed to try to get. None of those things provide the experience of the Real You. This makes it impossible for you to express your authentic Self while doing things not in alignment with your essence. What you do express, what you do share, is your mental, emotional, and societal conditioning, your EMI, and your subconscious programming.

The Most Persistent Cause of Suffering Is the Addiction to Identity

Cease to identify with roles, behaviors, concepts, beliefs, or the body. Cease to identify with anything and you will operate and express freely from the Real You. If you want to improve your life completely and utterly in every single way, start telling the truth. All your love, wisdom, talent, compassion, abilities, and power are the Real You. It is the only truth and the only way to be fully alive.

The subconscious, patterned, egoic mind is completely bankrupt and weak. It's easily knocked off its feet because it's not anchored to any tangible authenticity. All it takes is one bad text message, one bad report on the news, one unkind word from your partner, or one bad financial report and we freak out. Sometimes, all it takes is a look from someone and we lose it. That's how out of control, weak, and bankrupt the subconscious, patterned, egoic mind is. The Real You is unbreakable, invincible, and immortal.

The key to expressing the Real You is in giving up the programmed, personal agenda that you've capitulated your will and divinity to because of the hijacking of your mind. The Real You is the most powerful magnet for manifestation because the universe is optimally designed to mirror your highest vibration. And that core of you, of "what is," is connected to everything. The key to abundance in every facet of your life is to be completely aligned with the Real You. That is the magick of manifestation.

We must first deceive ourself before we deceive others. Start recognizing where you are fragmented, compartmentalized, and divided within yourself. There is no way to be the Real You when you are already lying to yourself. Remove your various personal agendas, and you cannot manipulate, coerce, or deceive others.

Metaphysically the only thing you're doing when you are not the Real You is constricting, collapsing, and fragmenting your own consciousness and energy. It leads to inauthenticity and limitation. The quality of your inner and outer life will reflect that. It's very difficult to be deceived once you stop deceiving yourself.

Effort-less Being-ness and Doing-ness

Being yourself takes no effort. Expressing your True Self takes no effort. As we stated earlier, a dog doesn't have to try to be a dog; it's a dog. You don't have to try to be yourself; you are yourself. All the effort is in trying to be something that you're not. This is no way to live or enjoy life. There is nothing "successful" in being well adjusted to a low-frequency, trauma-based, mind-controlled world society. In fact, it's the opposite. You have been profoundly diverted, completely inverted, and horribly perverted into various limitation programs. None of this is the Real You.

Clarity, calmness, connectivity, and communion is the nature of all existence. The goal is to work with yourself in this way. When you cease to divide, fragment, and compartmentalize yourself, every aspect of your life will reflect the fullness, connection, and unity of the One Self within us all. That unifying thread will be present in all moments. The Real You and your ability to express that authentically and perpetually will be yours once again.

As you continue to do the work outlined in this book, being true to yourself and expressing your True Self becomes the easiest thing in the world. Remember, if you're stressed out, it's because you're trying to be something that you're not. Don't deny what is in alignment with the Real You. Give up the various programmed agendas. There is no truth, authenticity, or Real You in any of that.

Every time you incarnate onto earth, or elsewhere for that matter, the goal is always the same: to tangibly experience your Self, realize the Self (Self-Realization), and express your Self. Experiencing the joy, love, wisdom, peace, power, connectivity, and communion with all life is the goal of every incarnation.

That is the nature of the one true concrete reality. To experience it, you must deprogram the fragmentation, compartmentalization, and separation that occurs through subconscious, egoic conditioning. To transcend these things is what a successful life is.

Give yourself permission to be the Real You. Ultimately, what the Self desires is its own presence—to feel its own completeness while having the human experience. Compassion, imagination, wisdom, love, and power flow when we're fully present. When you're not fully present, you only experience your conditioning perpetually draining your energy and contracting your consciousness.

Let life just happen because it's going to anyway. Learn to swim with the current, not against it. Allow all the infinite possible possibilities inherent within every moment to present themselves within the screen of your consciousness. Surrender to the ever-changing ebb and flow of existence itself and you can harness its power for your Self. Your life will transform when you start to adopt these things.

To expedite your ability to harness the current of existence for your growth and greater quality of life, you must understand, from a metaphysical perspective, the spiritual buzzword *acceptance*. Say the word *acceptance* to yourself and see what tangibly happens to your energy. There is a contraction. You can feel it. This is very important. All of us must understand the power of the words we say to ourselves and the spell they cast.

Let's look at this deeply. You may have been told to "accept" a situation, person, or behavior that may very well be wildly discordant to you. Do not. Ever. Just underneath acceptance is agreement. By accepting something wildly discordant, you are solidifying it by agreeing to it. You are saying to yourself that this is the one reality, and you are locking yourself into it. It certainly is not the one and only reality. All limitation is a product of the subconscious, patterned, egoic mind, and you are never locked into anything when you operate properly.

Acceptance is a lower-consciousness conditioned mindset that now requires huge energetic effort and straining, even for slight change, let alone total transformation. What you really are is your higher mind; you are your Higher Self—just less in volume. We are going to discover how to instantly shift into higher-mind metaphysics in an effortless way.

Now say the word *allowance*. Feel what happens to your energy. There is an expansion. This is also very important and tangible proof. By working with allowance, you are allowing the infinite possible possibilities to manifest themselves within the screen of your consciousness. You are no longer in agreement and locked into one perceived, discordant reality but rather open to the infinite sea of change and potential.

Allowance gives you the ability to receive greater awareness, greater possibilities, and a greater sense of Self. Allowance allows what is currently discordant to you to effortlessly shift and transmute its current condition. You are giving permission for that person, that condition, that situation—*life*—to flow because you have given yourself permission through allowance.

Here is a shortcut to let life flow out of your current accepted discordant, one-reality perception and into the infinite possible possibilities available within your higher mind. Never "spell yourself" again by avoiding the following seven words. Remember, with your Self-talk, the voice inside your head, you are literally putting a spell over your mind and body.

How

How shuts off your higher mind and forces a resultant lower-consciousness logic and linearity paradigm bound by space/time. It prevents transcendent and powerful inspiration and imagination from coming into your screen of consciousness. *How* foments effort, straining, and solidifies agreed upon limitations, and it is to be avoided at all costs.

Why

Asking *why* is one of the favorite pastimes of the patterned, subconscious, egoic mind. It arises to make "what is" fit within its accepted and agreed upon one-reality paradigm. Ultimately, *why* keeps you locked into the prison of reason through justification that forms your agreed upon, accepted, and discordant one reality.

Try

If we looked deeply at this word, we would realize, metaphysically speaking, it doesn't authentically exist. At the risk of sounding like Yoda from *Star Wars*, "Do or do not. There is no try." By simply removing the word *try* from your vocabulary, you will become ferociously efficient and far more effective in your endeavors.

Should

This is a powerful addiction born of the patterned, subconscious, egoic mind. *Should* happens due to the collapse of infinite possible possibilities at the behest of the accepted and agreed upon one-reality, even if it's totally unpalatable and discordant to the one doing the *shoulding*. There is no liberation, imagination, or transcendence in the realm of *should*.

Need

If you don't have it, then you don't need it. If you truly needed it, you'd already have it. The subconscious, egoic mind is never in the present moment. Therefore, it incessantly obsesses about what it needs as it relates to a past and future. Drop this word now and you will realize it's eternally not applicable and cannot serve your inevitable shift into greater Self-awareness and possible possibilities.

You don't need, ever. You certainly don't need to be right, validated, recognized, or entertained; you don't need to conquer or play the victim. That's the patterned, subconscious, egoic mind. Give up all the programmed agendas and fully love yourself—warts and all.

You can search this entire multiverse for eternity, and you will never ever find anyone more deserving of your love than you.

But

"But what about…" is the desire to keep reality closed. It nearly completely stifles your ability to shift into a more expansive state of awareness and therefore a better quality of life. Without this word, you will effectively eliminate your own internal stop sign that prevents the new roads that could appear within in your life.

Want

When you tangibly realize that everything is already within you, just as the tree is within the seedling, you will cease to disempower and delude yourself by using this word. *Want* keeps things out of reach as what you chase runs away. Implied within *want* is that what you seek is not currently available within your accepted and agreed upon one-reality. Shift to *allowance* and you will begin to feel that what you want is already a frequency currently contained within you.

For True Health, Your Body/Mind Must be Directly Attuned to the Real You

The human body was created and intended to take direction from the Real You, your True Self, and our universal cosmic consciousness. It cannot handle nor was it designed to take direction from the mental body (your subconscious, patterned, egoic mind) or emotional body. You tend to stay healthy, happy, and filled with vigor and vitality when directing and experiencing your life from the Real You.

When you operate in alignment with the Real You, there's a tangible quality to this inner harmony. There's almost no activity that goes on in the rational/thinking mind or in the emotional body. Thinking (not knowing) and emoting (not loving) are replaced with knowing (intuitive wisdom) and loving (unconditional compassion and joy).

This is the perpetual flow state or being "in the zone" all the time. Another word for the flow state would be *meditation*, and you could even say another higher-consciousness aspect of that would be unbounded imagination and channeling. Everything pure flows through the Real You because the Real You is everything.

To be (or not to be) and express the Real You, you must first be present. In other words, not thinking. You may say to yourself and others that you have a very busy and hectic life, that if you don't think about everything, your life will fall apart. That notion is just a belief, and a belief is nothing more than a string of thoughts. Whatever "falls apart" means you have outgrown it and it no longer serves your highest good.

How Non-Thought Relates to Your Health

As we stated earlier, the physical body was designed for optimum health and longevity when you operate in alignment with the Real You. One way you can tap into this immediately is allowing yourself to become completely engrossed in something—full and total and engagement in what you're doing.

What you're doing is irrelevant. What is of paramount importance is that you're completely engaged and engulfed in what you're doing. This is what it means to "lose yourself" in something. What you are losing is the subconscious, patterned, egoic mind—the false Self.

Whether it's having a conversation, playing a board game or a sport, cooking, dancing, writing, painting, making love, washing the dishes, it doesn't matter. Recall when you've been completely and utterly engaged in what you're doing. Start to recall the energetic quality of what it's like when you're totally engaged, when you've lost yourself in what you're doing.

Notice that there's no thought process. This is a surefire way to know that you are expressing, engaging, and being the Real You. That flow state, meditative state, channeling state, pure creative state are all aspects of the exact same thing: being and expressing the Real You.

Conversely, when you lead a life where the thoughts, actions, and behaviors are directed from the mental or emotional body, it, too, has a tangible quality to it. Examine where in your body you feel these directives coming from. That will give you proof as to their origination point, meaning they do not belong or come from the Real You.

Recall what it feels like when you have an onerous responsibility to something or someone. You're doing it out of a sense of responsibility due to an indentation or identification regarding some concept, belief, or role. Feel what it's like when you "must" do something. It doesn't feel right. It feels heavy and you feel off, and hence you feel uncomfortable. This is proof that you're not expressing or being the Real You.

The Real You is perfect, whole, and complete. The Real You doesn't suffer. The mind/body suffers when the subconscious, patterned EMI is leading the incarnation. But as we alluded to previously, the sun is untouched by the clouds and severe weather. You, the Real You, are untouched by the body/mind complex. It doesn't matter what's going on with the body/mind; it never touches you. The key is to align the body/mind with the Real You. That is how to express the Real You.

Express the Real You versus Subconscious, Patterned, Egoic Programming

Let's go back to when you're not being/expressing the Real You. There is a recognition of mental, emotional, and/or physical stress and disharmony. You know exactly what this feels like. The Real You does not create nor experience this—ever. It is untouchable, unscathed, and unaffected.

The programmed human character is always seeking something because it is imbalance and disharmony itself. The Real You is perpetually at equilibrium, in harmony, and joyous. The programmed mind must seek everything out, figure everything out, including health, because it's utterly bankrupt and inauthentic. Start to see the difference between these two things.

When you're being and expressing the Real You, it's an effortless free flow. Pure imagination is the play of the higher mind. It has a meditative quality to it. That is because the flow state is frequentially above thinking and emoting. The Real You is effortless alignment, and therefore, you become fully engaged in whatever you're doing.

Conversely, you experience constant struggle to remain in servitude to the programmed mind. That's how you tangibly know you're not being/expressing the Real You. There is no flow. It's not natural. There's a weight to mentally and emotionally driven behavior. You can feel it. With it comes the stress of forced effort to achieve, acquire, or become what you already are beneath the layers of programming.

As we discovered earlier, if you're stressed, it means you're trying to be something that you're not or you are in denial of what is. Really examine the truth of this regarding your energy and state of being. Take stock of the difference when you're being and expressing the Real You as opposed to when these other things are occurring.

Examine why you're doing it. You'll find some deep-rooted programming (belief/indentation/identification with a role, form, concept, image, ideology, or memory), and you're either trying to live up to it, fix what isn't in alignment with it, or make amends using it.

Awareness of Your Human Character's Motivation

As you recognize these things within you, don't disregard them. Investigate them. Go to the root cause. Understand your true motivation. Ask yourself, "Why am I doing this? What is it that I feel right now? Why do I think this way? Why do I feel uncomfortable? Why am I starting to get anxious, depressed, or aggressive? Why do I feel depleted, defeated, or depressed?" Examining and understanding the outer human personality are the keys to being/expressing the Real You.

Another one of the keys to expressing the Real You is to live a life in accordance with your passions. Work with what excites you and what you're truly interested in. We've all heard the saying, "Do what you love, and you'll never work a day in your life." It's true. See life as play and your life will be a joy.

Move your awareness and focus to where your passions reside, to your highest excitement. When in alignment, you will be excited to wake up in the morning and for what the day has in store for you or, more accurately, for what you are going to infuse that day with.

Allow yourself to tangibly remember what it felt like when you were much younger. Feel it. Now remember what you were really excited about. Maybe it was baseball, music, exercising, caring for animals, writing, travel, etc. Whatever it was, simply recall when you were seriously passionate about it and truly interested in it. Tangibly remember that you couldn't wait to do it! That resonance is the key to being/expressing the Real You.

Through the teachings of this book, I want you to rediscover that feeling daily. From moment to moment, be truly engaged and aware and awake. This is truly being alive! Live your greatest potential at your highest excitement. Rediscover what your deepest passions are because that's the Real You experiencing/expressing the depth of itself. This world—and you—need it desperately.

That is how to live authentically—by expressing and sharing the depth of yourself. Let your love, wisdom, joy, passion, talents, and abilities flow. You can never run out of these things because they are you. It's not possible to run out of love and wisdom. It's just the opposite. The more you share it, the more you are experiencing it yourself.

Allow your highest excitement to move you. Let joy rule. Genuine excitement and acceptance are your new default settings. That's when you know you're being and expressing the Real You. If you're in a relationship that doesn't allow you to do that, then that's a relationship (either your own Self-talk or regarding a partner) that needs to be examined.

The right relationship, business, circumstance, environment, activities, group of friends, people—the right you name it—will foster your highest potential and joy, not stifle it, hold it down, limit it, or compartmentalize, judge, or discourage it.

Give Yourself Permission to Be and Express the Real You

Utilize the teachings in the book to experience the greatest quality of life. Dedicate yourself so you can always operate as the Real You with passion, excitement, and love. Through living this way, you will tap into your indomitable will and greatest purpose. They go hand in hand because the purpose is to release and share these aspects of the Real You. When you align the body/mind with the Real You, you will realize you can accept and overcome any obstacle or challenge with grace.

Remember, freedom has no meaning without purpose, and your purpose is to be and express the Real You.

Live your life with tremendous passion, fierce determination, great purpose, unconditional love, an open mind, and a forgiving heart. Infuse every moment with these qualities of the Real You. Infuse your entire body and body of energy with that excitement, passion, and wisdom. That is a life worth living. That is a life worth sharing. That is a life worth fighting for.

Summary

To be fully engaged, totally present, and completely engulfed in whatever you are doing is how to express and experience the Real You. When you "lose yourself" in the moment, what you are losing—from a pure physics perspective—is the electro/magnetic/interference, or the EMI, along with its shadow: your patterned, subconscious mind. You only lose what you are not. The state of unification with being-ness and doing-ness is how to express the Real You.

The "what" you do, including the absence of physical, mental, or emotional doing, does not stop the expression of the Real You. The Real You is online when unification or a flow state is tangibly experienced. The Real You, your true vibration, is broadcast even in the absence of what you would typically label as doing. This is unfiltered emanation, sans your electro/magnetic/interference, and is the direct expression of the Real You.

Expressing the Real You does not require thought, approval, validation, permission, attention, or analysis. Those are habits born of the conditioned mind. Your joy, excitement, and passion have nothing to do with the conditioned mind. In fact, you feel those qualities through expressing the Real You only when they are absent. The Real You is the ultimate, unbreakable, and eternal permission slip to express your true nature now and forever.

Let the Real You flow unabated into, through, and with every moment. Feel the Real You expressing itself continually and without effort. Give it voice, feeling, and action! Let it dance upon the stage of this world. The Real You is a polyphonic symphony expressing itself in physical form. There are no auditions, my friend. You have already been cast as the star, director, and producer. So quiet on the set (meditation)! Lights (the Real You present)! Camera (ever-expanding awareness)! Action (limitless creative expression)!

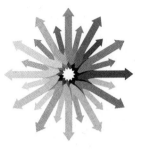

Chapter 6
Universal Characteristics of the Real You

Let's take a deeper look at these universal aspects or qualities of the Real You. Here are the top thirteen qualities and attributes of the Real You that you must express in order to be happy and fulfilled.

#1: Patience

Wisdom flowers within the soil of patience. Being in harmony with the eternal flow of the Self will naturally engender patience. The Self is presence and awareness. It is immortal. It is beyond space/time and therefore never in a rush or running late. Let everything unfold in your life by always resting within the patience born of true immortality.

When you are engaged in a conversation with anyone, listen to them without thinking or worrying about formulating a response.

#2: Talents and Abilities

The Real You is love and wisdom, and its subsets are what we call talents and abilities. Recognizing what you are drawn to, excited and passionate about will often bring out your natural talents and abilities. We come into the world with inherent talents and abilities because they are part of what we are. Let your interest, excitement, and passion bring out what is already within you.

Make the time every day to create something that is near and dear to your heart and give it away. It can be anything you like to create, such as a meal, a drawing, a song, an email, or a nugget of wisdom from personal experience that you share with someone or something that needs it.

#3: Determination

The energy you use to think, emote, and animate the body is your will. Focusing your will gives you true willpower. This is determination. Always keeping your word builds great determination. Once you learn not to suffer even small defeats about keeping your word, you will soon have strengthened your will sufficiently to overcome anything because you have learned how to harness true willpower (determination).

When you wake up in the morning, ask yourself what it is that you would really like to do today. Once you determine what that is, make a promise to yourself that you will do it today, and do not break your promise to yourself. It could be to clean the garage, to meditate, to go for a walk, anything really. Just do not break your promise to yourself. This strengthens your will and gives you formidable determination in life.

#4: Joy

Joy is part of the very fabric of the Real You. Never question, contain, or limit your joy. That is like being the warden of your very own Self-imposed prison. Let joy—the Real You—carry you through the vicissitudes of life. Joy never ceases to flow because it is you.

Every day, do something that truly brings you joy. Remember that feeling is inside you; it is you. Sometimes we need a permission slip to bring it out. Maybe watch a movie that makes you laugh, engage in a game with a friend or roommate, or play with your companion entity.

#5: Acceptance

Within the screen of your consciousness, there is nothing to reject, hold on to, or chase. The Real You is full acceptance, sans any internal dialogue. Acceptance of the Self is only possible through being present. The Real You is so incomprehensibly unlimited, immeasurably spacious, and so unconditionally loving that it has room for everything and everyone—starting with you. Acceptance provides the knowingness that everything and everyone gets to evolve in their own way and in their own time.

Pretend that you just arrived here—no past, no future. Let your mind become so still that the play of all life is directly and tangibly experienced. Do not let the egoic mind take over. Just experience the play of life with no analysis, no expectation, and no rumination.

#6: Wisdom

The recognition of inner knowingness is wisdom. Your wisdom is already and eternally present. It is you. Wisdom does not take the form of thought or intellectualism but rather predates and can give birth to them. Wisdom is timeless and therefore goes beyond the contextual meanderings and limitation of intellectualism. We only think about what we don't know; we never think about what we already tangibly know to be true.

Writing is the geometry of the Soul. It brings your wisdom into conscious view. Self-reflect by journaling on how you spent your energy (the thoughts, emotions, actions, and behaviors). Did you spend your day thinking and about what? Examine it through journaling. Self-reflect on your being-ness while interacting with people. Were you kind, pushy, compassionate, short-tempered, loving, articulate?

#7: Contentment

Being at peace no matter the circumstance is a hallmark of the Real You. Think of a perfectly balanced scale. The Real You is eternally balanced and harmonious because the concepts of "lack and excess" do not exist within the Real You. Those experiences belong to the patterned, subconscious, egoic mind. Where ying meets yang is the eternal contentment of the Real You.

Every day, turn off your disharmonious, egoic mind and lose yourself in the play of nature. For example, sit under a tree and watch birds nesting, waves crashing, dogs playing, squirrels gathering nuts, or fish swimming.

#8: Creativity

We are immortal creator beings. We feel most like ourselves when we are creating. What you create is irrelevant if the inspiration flows directly from the Real You, not the subconscious, patterned, egoic mind. When you operate this way, what you give birth to through the act of creation will be imbued with the depth of your love and wisdom.

Every day, tell yourself a story about you—your character—that captures your own triumph and victory over any obstacle. It doesn't matter what story or stories you create as long as they're reflective of the Real You.

#9: Spontaneity

Unlike the patterned, egoic mind, the Real You has no habits. That is because what you really are is formless, free, and unconditioned. Living in the now and thus being spontaneous is the truest and best way to live. Remove as many habitual behaviors as possible and you will give rise to the eternal freshness, unlimited potential, and spontaneity of the Real You.

Without planning, whatever you are most excited about doing in the moment, do it. This is one way to remember what it's like to be free of the programmed mind.

#10: Purpose

The Real You is impelled with a purpose that goes beyond the individual. This purpose does not come from mere mental or emotional stimulation. It is birthed from up on high and infuses your very being. Every notion we give birth to ideally will be filled with a purpose that goes well beyond the limitations of the body/mind complex. This higher purpose is God working through you, as you, within you, and for you.

Ask yourself, "What is the single most important driving force in my life?" Is it something outside of yourself, like another person, a belief, or your temporary physical body? True purpose already exists and was determined by the Real You well before any of those things became manifest. With that as your new understanding, ask yourself what the single most important driving force in your life is. Are you serving it with love, kindness, unbreakable will, and acceptance?

#11: Forgiveness

Being able to take each moment as it comes, unencumbered by the concepts of past/future, allows the flower of compassion to infuse the mind with the aroma of forgiveness. By forgiving, we allow ourselves to fully experience the majesty, fullness, and richness of every now. Forgiveness starts within by releasing all Self-judgment. Once we do that, our heart opens and no ill will or fear can ever be broadcast or received.

#12: Love

Love, which is unconditional, is the summation of all wisdom. The Real You, ultimately, is unconditional love. Give your current incarnation the gift of love and your life will be transmuted into joy. The vibration of unconditional love emanates and reverberates throughout all space/time and is the most powerful force that births all existence. Every day, do something that comes directly from your heart (not mind) and stay attuned to that feeling all day and all night.

#13: Gratitude

Incarnation is such a gift. It is full of wonder and a bottomless treasure. The magnificence of physical reality cannot be captured by the machinations of the finite mind or mere bodily sensations. Do not overvalue what you do not have and undervalue what you do have. The vibration of gratitude will envelop you and raise your frequency.

To experience true gratitude use "Thank You" as a mantra. Connect with the words and say them again and again. Watch what happens.

Summary

The thirteen universal characteristics of the Real You are ways for you to experience more of what you eternally are. The subconscious, patterned, egoic mind is conditioned and programmed to operate with the implicit acceptance directive that everything lies outside of the Self. The fact is these universal characteristics are aspects or qualities of your eternal essence. Nothing must be done to acquire them. Rather, we must surrender and cultivate what is already contained within.

We are encouraged to lose all tangible connection to our own universal and inherent completeness. The truth about ourselves is not cultivated within our low-frequency world culture. Instead, we are "educated" on how to memorize, obey authority, and not think for ourselves. We are programmed to perform tasks, fit in, color inside the lines, and limit and separate ourselves through identifications. We are taught how to spell ourselves and each other, but we are not taught what it takes to be happy, loving, wise, and free.

The good news is that these internal aspects of us just need to be reawakened. They are you. Through these simple insights, we can delete what has kept us misaligned and unhappy. The Real You is always aware of everything that is going on. It's time to be consciously creating your life instead of watching your conditioned mind obey and react to it.

Dedicate the changing of your mind to the liberation of your joy, creativity, and happiness. Let your life be an expression of the timelessness and eternal beauty of your Soul. Marinate within these universal characteristics and let them bubble over into this world—into your world. This life is a gift, and like all gifts, it's best when shared.

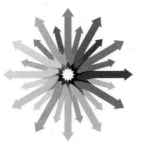

Chapter 7

Activities to Integrate
the Real You in Everyday Life

In the previous chapter, we learned about the thirteen universal characteristics of the Real You. In this chapter, you are going to discover activities and exercises that incorporate them into your everyday life. You do not need to infuse your life with detailed or complicated protocols to bring magick back into your life. By being yourself, your True Self, and performing these fun activities and easy exercises, you can feel the magick already in you.

The activities that reintegrate the Real You into your everyday life have nothing to do with needing fancy technology, lots of money, or an abundance of resources. They require no advanced degrees, extensive travel, profound worldly experience, or even help from anyone. This is important to take note of. You always have and eternally are what you have always sought.

Remember, if you're stressed, anxious, or depressed, it's because you're trying to be someone or something that you're not. It's the expectations programmed in or that we have chosen to identify with that causes us to suffer. It is our misperceptions, misunderstandings, and misidentifications that constitute our patterned, subconscious, egoic mind. Without those things, you are free, and these exercises give you back the tangible experience of the Real You.

Change Your Mind:
13 Days of Activities to Awaken the Real You

Being in alignment with the Real You at first may feel strange. That's because the conditioned, egoic mind has been driving the bus of this incarnation. In no time—in fact, in just under two weeks—you will have grabbed a hold of the wheel of your life! Now the journey and destination are truly up to you!

Note: The full and permanent integration of the feeling and state of consciousness you experience while engaged in these activities is the key. Make the integration of the Real You ongoing and perpetual rather than something limited by an activity or duration. Carry and continually experience that greater sense of Self into and in every moment moving forward. That greater and expanded state is simply more and more of the Real You.

Add and incorporate the feeling and state of consciousness from the previous days into the next day and its activity. The fullness of the Real You never runs dry, goes away, or can ever be used up. It is the eternal life force itself and you are it.

Day #1: Patience

Have a conversation with someone without interrupting them or thinking about formulating a response while they are speaking. Take time to perform an activity that promotes patience, such as fishing, gardening, writing, or assembling a puzzle.

Day #2: Talents and Abilities

Make time today to create something that is near and dear to your heart and give it away. It can be anything: a meal, a drawing, a hand-written letter, etc.

Day #3: Determination

Make a promise to yourself when you wake up and do it that very day. It could be to clean the garage, to meditate, to go for a walk, to take a drive, or to call a loved one. Set the intention and follow through.

Day #4: Joy

You are joy. Sometimes you need to break your habitual patterns in order to give yourself the permission slip needed to bring it out! Laugh and play with your grandchildren, relatives, siblings, parents, coworkers, companion entities, friends, etc.

Day #5: Acceptance

Let the mind become so still that the ebb and flow of all life is directly and tangibly experienced. No analysis, no expectation, no rumination. Meditate, do yoga, stretch, lose yourself in pure observation, and breathe deeply from the diaphragm.

Day #6: Wisdom

Reflect by journaling on how you spent your energy today (thoughts, emotions, actions, and behaviors). Did you spend your day thinking/doing, and about what? Reflect on how you behaved while interacting with people. Were you kind, pushy, short-tempered, determined, attentive, etc.?

Day #7: Contentment

Turn off your egoic mind and lose yourself in the play of nature. Sit under a tree and watch waves crash onto the shore or observe dogs playing, birds flying, squirrels gathering nuts, or fish swimming.

Day #8: Creativity

Make something—anything. It doesn't matter as long as it's reflective of the Real You. Draw, paint, cook or bake, write a song or poem, plant a flower, write an email, dance, create an online course, write a fantasy short story, make a collage, etc.

Day #9: Spontaneity

Without planning, whatever you are most excited about doing in the moment, simply do it. This is one way to remember what it's like to be free of the programmed mind. Go to that movie you have wanted to see, the museum, or the farmers' market. Go see your friend or relative, take a balloon ride, ride go karts, attend a sports game, go on a day trip, start your miniature garden, etc.

Day #10: Purpose

Ask yourself, "What is the single most important driving force in my life?" Once you have your answer, do something today that you have never done in service to that. Use your imagination. Don't think outside the box—remove the box—and make it happen!

Day #11: Forgiveness

Beginning today and moving forward, look in the mirror and say to yourself, "I forgive you." Mean it when you say it. Say it ten times, sincerely, and watch what happens.

Day #12: Love

Love is the most powerful vibration in all existence. It dismantles and destroys everything other than itself. Give something away, whether it is your time, a gift, energy, money, food, a family heirloom, know-how, and neither expect nor accept anything in return. Make the gift something that comes directly from your heart that you know someone needs and would appreciate. Take yourself out of the equation. Stay attuned to this feeling all day and all night.

Day #13: Gratitude

Deep appreciation or gratitude for "what is" is full presence in the now. Make "Thank You" your mantra. Connect with the words and say them again and again. Watch what happens. Pure magick!

Bonus Change Your Mind: 48-Hour Retreat Tips to Accelerate Meeting the Real You!

One fun and effective way to deprogram the subconscious, patterned, egoic mind is by removing yourself from your familiar surroundings. Familiarity breeds comfort and the subconscious, patterned, egoic mind is built upon what it is familiar with—even if what's familiar is very uncomfortable, upsetting, or stressful.

Although not necessary, going camping by the local river, getting a hotel room, or even renting an Airbnb for the weekend is a fantastic way to set yourself up for success while doing your forty-eight-hour challenge if you can leave home.

While you will still follow the guidelines of chapter 3's notebook challenge during your forty-eight-hour retreat, here are the top four ways to accelerate, condense, and supercharge your subconscious deprogramming to meet the Real You!

Turn Off Your Phone!

Turning off your phone/computer removes the primary distractions (technology) that keep you from truly getting to know the Real You. In a section of your notebook, keep track of all the times you unconsciously reach for your phone to scroll, research, shop, post, message someone, or take a photo. Write it down and question why you are really doing it.

No Television

Most of us use TV/movie watching to numb, procrastinate, distract, or entertain ourselves rather than get to know our own completeness, resourcefulness, creativity, and ever-present inner peace and love. Instead of TV watching, practice meditation and notebook the thoughts/emotions that arise from within the subconscious, patterned, egoic mind. You can even inquire if some of those identifications/beliefs were things that you simply bought into because you saw them on television/online.

Get a Mirror

This is not for you to obsess over your hair, worry about a wrinkle, or panic because of a blemish. Instead, each day I want you to stand in front of a mirror (or hold one in your hand), look yourself in the eyes, and say "I AM the conqueror of my mind and body." Say it ten times.

You must look into your eyes, connect with yourself, and mean it when you say, "I AM the conqueror of my mind and body." Whatever thoughts or emotions arise from this, notebook them and drill down on them like an archaeologist digging for a lost buried treasure (the Real You!).

Go On a Nature Walk

Moving your body while connecting with nature is an elixir for grounding, rejuvenation, and purification. Take in the beauty and wonder of your natural surroundings. As your state of being and thought patterns begin to change, stop and notebook what comes to you. Exercising and notebooking in nature gives you the permission to stop focusing on what's at the forefront of your patterned, subconscious, egoic mind. This gives you a wonderful opportunity to deprogram. Take advantage of it while reconnecting with your own true nature.

Summary

When we look carefully from a higher-consciousness perspective at the activities that integrate the Real You, we see that they each have one immutable and eternal commonality. They all represent the total absence of electro/magnetic/interference (EMI) or the subconscious, patterned, egoic mind. These activities are the physical expression or pure flow state that is the Real You.

In essence, by performing these activities, you have learned how to get out of your way. The disruptive electrical current of our subconscious, patterned, egoic mind is the only resistance that exists. From this experience of resistance, blocks and obstacles are tangibly felt and therefore believed in. Thus, they become "real" and we subsequently spell ourselves into the reality of impossibility through our Self-talk.

Marry yourself to the experience of these activities through repetition. We get highly proficient at what we do repetitively. The goal is to never divorce your body/mind from how you feel when you perform them. Now, these qualities are permanently felt. Eventually, you will find every activity you perform will be an expression of the Real You.

Part of the instantaneous efficacy of the forty-eight-hour challenge is owed to the removal of electronics. When we remove our brain and body of energy from the effects of their frequencies, we immediately begin to align to our own vibration. Do not underestimate the immense transformative and rejuvenative power of true communion with nature. It is you and you are it—directly. Surrender to the high-frequency electrical current of what is, and all your seeking will finally come to end.

Part 3
Attending to Your Energy

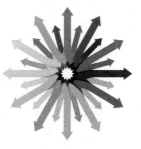

Chapter 8

Balance Your Energy
Bank Account

In terms of your temporary experience as a human being, you use energy for everything. It's the gas in the gas tank, so to speak. What you may not realize is that it's your chakra system that receives and metabolizes your life force energy, not food.

What you really are is sentience (divine intelligence—love and wisdom whose subsets are talents and abilities) given an allotment or complement of energy (sentience + energy = Total Self) to create with. This is universal for all sentient beings on this planet and elsewhere.

You use energy to think, emote, animate the body, and create experiences. Without the energy you are given, you would essentially be inert and unable to create. Imagine being locked into a state of non-animation and non-functionality. Being permanently paralyzed is a good analogy, and I am quite familiar with "permanent paralysis" and the metaphysics required to transcend it. These higher-consciousness teachings, understandings, and protocols are captured in my first book, *Supercharged Self-Healing*, along with countless stories of others who radically improved their health and state of being.

In the preceding chapters, you learned a great deal about how your energetic bedspread (projected by your subconscious mind) is affected by indentations and identifications. Your body of energy is massively impacted from the stimulus your five senses perceive, but it is also greatly affected by subtle phenomena outside physical sensory perception.

Your energy—how it is affected and how you use it—dictates your entire quality of life. Because you use energy for everything, it is paramount that you are masterful with perception, play, use, and control of your energy. Nothing is more important than you learning to master your energy and, eventually, other energies.

How to Spend Your Most Precious Resource Wisely

Because you have a limited or finite amount of energy to work with during a single lifetime, being wise regarding its usage is of supreme importance. As we have talked about previously, your subconscious, patterned, egoic mind has dictated how you've spent your most precious commodity: your life force. Now that you have a deep, tangible understanding of how to effectively deprogram your conditioned and egoic mind, you are changing your mind and your life.

If you have a location that you need to get to and you have decided that specific destination is your highest priority, it would be foolish to make extraneous pit stops along the way. When you do so, you are using up your limited gas for excursions that are not paramount to you, and you may not have enough gas left for what is most important.

Being mindful—masterful—with how you spend your energy will greatly elevate and enhance your entire quality of life. You may find that you often procrastinate or distract yourself. These unnecessary pit stops drain your life force by vampirizing your energy. It is vital that you summon the will to focus on what you have deemed a priority. Attention is energy, and you only have so much of it. Don't ever waste it. Ever.

Your energetic bank account is debited by everything you give attention to. That is why it's called *paying* attention. Every phenomenon you pay attention to grows. You, on the other hand, become depleted and less flush with your most precious commodity. Start seeing your attention (energy) as the greatest resource you own. Treat it with the utmost respect and hold it in the highest regard. Energy is the Holy Ghost.

Can We Refuel and Increase Our Energy?

The question regarding how to summon and increase my energy was a crucial component in my Self-healing journey to overcome "permanent" chest-down paralysis, severe illnesses, and life-threatening conditions. I discovered, or remembered, really, how to command and channel powerful high-frequency energy into my body. It became a matter of tapping into the proper energy source and formulating a robust, repeatable, and efficient process.

Where you and I are right now—the low frequencies of the physical universe—it is nearly inevitable that we'll become immersed and attached to things here. Subsequently, you lose energy (through *paying* attention and possible attachment) rather than gain it. Our local environment is extremely low and sticky. It drains your gas tank.

Without your new understanding of metaphysics and how to deprogram the subconscious mind through the simple yet profoundly effective notebook exercise, you would perpetually spill your most precious commodity with little to no meaningful return on your investments. The only tangible and meaningful return is the evolution of your immortal Soul, not your human character.

Before we get into the mechanics and application of your energy diagnostic system, let's take look at this expansive landscape from a significantly higher-consciousness perspective.

The Most Precious Resource

How are you to locate and subsequently spend your most precious resource (attention) on the single investment opportunity that always yields the greatest and only true return on investment. Knowing what to do, whom to mix your energy with, and what pursuits are most worthwhile is priceless. Knowing whom and what to avoid is just as valuable. There is a supreme investment opportunity available, and we are going to discover it right now.

What is the only thing that endures? Not your mind/body complex, not empires, dynasties, or physical possessions, and certainly not your beliefs, concepts, stock portfolio, or expectations. What is it that cocreates all phenomenon, lifetime after lifetime? It's the Immortal Self: the Real You.

The divine creator within, by utilizing its most precious and heavenly resource (energy), gives birth to every incarnation. It is the only thing that endures. So, why not go all in on the only thing that eternally remains? Why not cut out the middleperson, your subconscious, patterned, egoic mind and all its delusions, and invest directly in the Real You?

Afraid of what you will lose by investing? It is your ignorance and arrogance that you perpetually suffer from that will finally be lost forever. The subconscious, patterned, egoic mind that fears loss and craves acquiring is the tangible experience of the unawakened mind. Your delusional and bankrupt subconscious, patterned, egoic mind authentically owns nothing, which is why it clings to things. Fear, greed, and restlessness rob you of your most precious resource (energy), stealing your inner equilibrium, power, timeless wisdom, eternal freedom, unconditional love, unending joy, and lasting peace.

Energetic thievery, always done at the behest of your subconscious, patterned, egoic mind, is caught red-handed and finally handcuffed by the protocols and teachings within this book. Consciously driven imagination, true joy, and palpable empowerment are tangibly known and back with their rightful owner when you adhere to these teachings. The fear of failure, success, loss, and lack will float away along with the patterned, subconscious, egoic mind that produced it.

A New Paradigm

Stop deluding yourself into thinking your outside world will change by analyzing it. That's an investment strategy that will only perpetuate your suffering. Constant analysis, compartmentalization, and fragmentation are all symptoms of internal disempowerment. Stop leaking all your power, wisdom, and courage on the very same illusions that your patterned, subconscious, egoic mind belongs to.

If you cannot figure out how to invest directly in the Real You, your experience in this life will be a perpetual, unsatisfying struggle at best and a catastrophic nightmare at worst. This book is a teleporter out of that abyss. If your commitment to liberation is not followed up with the expenditure of tangible and intangible resources, then you have not made a commitment at all. One does not test-drive the evolution of consciousness. It isn't something to dabble in like a start-up, psychedelics, a new concept, or a get-rich-quick scheme.

Investment requires skin in the game. You are incarnate now, so your human character has everything to gain and absolutely nothing to lose except its own suffering and karma. Your subconscious programming prevents the experience of true freedom and liberation. All the concepts, hopes, beliefs, bodily experiences, and expectations you have invested in yield only a greater appetite for more temporary phenomena. More prisons for the body/mind. More suffering.

When you pursue the desires, praise the vanity, avoid the fears, and seek the pleasures of the subconscious, patterned, egoic mind, you are utilizing what appears to be your free will. Your free will—your energy—has been stolen by low-frequency subconscious programming and egoic identifications. This is what societal conditioning and brainwashing are. You are now under their spell, and your every thought, emotion, action, and behavior are always done at the behest of your patterned mind, which is totally controlled by and belongs to the vast matrix of low-frequency illusion.

You cannot escape from the matrix until you see and admit that you are the matrix. You have trapped yourself in time by thinking. By creating a past and future through thought, you have lost the Real You and become a mere shadow blocking your own light. You only serve your indentations and identifications, not your love, evolution, and ascension. All purely humanistic desires, fears, and bodily sensations are not worthwhile investments. These pursuits and endeavors are catastrophically the worst investments of your most precious resource—energy.

When does the investment of your attention do anything other than keep you imprisoned within the sensory realm? Your temporary satiation of purely human desires, the panic-driven need for security, or the momentarily quelling of your fear are all produced by your unawakened mind. Is this not an investment strategy that should be avoided at all costs since it yields nothing but more craving and addictions? It's not a bad investment strategy; it's the metaphysical definition of insanity.

If you have no tangible and direct experience of the Real You, then you can never choose the right investment. Is this why "civilized" society is perpetually inundated with stimulus? Delusion, division, and destruction by distraction. Phenomena, by definition, is that which comes and goes, and therefore, it is unreliable at best and a literal illusion at worst. All poor investments from any perspective. Politics, entertainment, technology, intellectualism, information, beliefs, concepts, physical goods, experiences, ideologies, so-called knowledge, all sensory realm phenomena… What of this endures? What is the way out of the endless cycle of suffering through rebirth and death we call samsara?

The Wisdom That Transcends Knowledge

Processing stimulus through the conditioned analytical mind only delays your own liberation and peace. Then how do you invest your energy directly in the one thing that endures, that is real, that yields the perpetual flowering of love, wisdom, and power?

You must question the behaviors and notions that consume your energy. Discover your true motivation behind your every notion. That is power. You cannot deeply invest your most precious resource—energy—until you do so first. Use the teachings and protocols outlined in this book to guide you. As you uncover the subconscious, patterned, egoic mind, stay present with your newfound realizations and epiphanies. Let them become tangibly known within your heart. This is gnosis.

As you remove the indentations and identifications, allow yourself to fall in love with your own inner stillness and silence. Marry yourself to the seemingly silent yet polyphonic symphony of existence through surrender. Know that if you are reading this book, our well-planned meeting (once again) has come to fruition.

It's time to put the toys away. They may very well be taken from you anyway. Now you can begin investing your greatest resource—attention—into the limitless inner expansion of the only thing that brings everlasting dividends: the Real You.

Change Your Mind: Run Your Energy Diagnostic Tests

Once you have freed yourself from the tyranny of your subconscious, patterned, egoic mind, the question becomes how to always get the best return on your most valuable investment—your attention. As we discussed earlier, attention is energy. Where your attention goes, your energy flows. Knowing what gives the best return on your investment of attention is paramount to a happy, fulfilling, successful, purposeful, and joyous life.

You have discovered that certain people, things, and activities sometimes leave you drained, stressed, or exhausted. That can come in the form of feeling less positive about yourself, a little frazzled emotionally or mentally, not quite right physically, or even all the way to feeling like you just encountered an energy vampire. This planet is rife with them.

You have also experienced that certain people, things, and activities rejuvenate you. There are some people who truly lift your spirits. You feel happier, empowered, more centered, and lighter after engaging with them. You look forward to these encounters, and often you form a friendship or a relationship or have business transactions with them.

Often though, you may find yourself unsure about getting involved with a certain person, circumstance, business, activity, group, or event. You have mixed feelings because you can see both the potential benefits and pitfalls. I have discovered a simple, repeatable, and robust way to shed light on this problem.

From a metaphysical perspective, there is no good or bad, right or wrong, positive or negative. Those are truly subjective. What is objective is high frequency or low frequency. This can be proven by the tangible effect upon your well-being. Now, finally, this can be measured and quantified with your new energy diagnostic system.

How It Works

By asking yourself a series of five simple yet illuminating questions prior to engaging, during engagement, and post engagement, you will record your answers. Each answer will be tallied on a scoring system that goes from zero to five.

At the end of each series of five questions, you will tally your points. The result will be a tangible and objective answer as to whether it cost you energy and/or drop your frequency or revitalized you and/or raised your frequency. Simple, powerful, effective, and illuminating.

With your new revolutionary, effective energy diagnostic system, you will know if the return on investment, or ROI, of your most precious asset (energy in the form of your attention) was worth the expenditure. You are going to use your energy diagnostic system for three separate categories:

- Activities
- People
- Circumstances/events

There are four ways a human being can express itself: emotionally, mentally, verbally, and physically. You are going to use these fundamental forms of expression to measure your state of being before, during, and after your engagement.

To assess your purely energetic state of being, you will use your inner voice or Real You to capture that data. Get ready because what you are about to discover on how you spend your most precious resource—attention—will change your entire life.

What You Need

You can either create a note on your smartphone, computer, or tablet; use your notebook from your notebook exercise; or get a brand-new notebook. I suggest using a brand-new notebook for your energy diagnostic system. Divide your notebook (or electronic note) into the three separate categories of activities, people, and circumstances/events.

What It Looks Like

Before engaging, write down:

- How do I feel emotionally leading up to…?
- What is my thought process leading up to…?
- How do I feel energetically (inner voice) leading up to…?
- How do I feel physically leading up to…?

During engagement, include:

- How do I feel emotionally during…?
- What is my thought process during…?
- How do I feel energetically (inner voice) while engaged…?
- How do I feel physically while engaged…?

Post engagement, write down:

- How do I feel emotionally after…?
- What is my thought process after…?
- How do I feel energetically (inner voice) after…?
- How do I feel physically after…?

These short but illuminating written answers will give you tremendous insight into your state of being. They will also clarify your entire experience in an entirely new way. You will no longer walk away after some form of engagement not fully aware and mindful of what you brought to the table, how you engaged, and what your tangible take away was.

Balancing Your Energy Bank Account

You are now ready to calculate your energetic scoring. The ultimate purpose is to discover how to always maintain a positive flow into your energy bank account. Recognizing and quantifying what empowers or disempowers you is essential in the quality of life you experience. It also paves the way for your new unleashed ability to create your life as you deem fit. Attention (energy) is your most precious and sacred resource. You are about to learn how to spend it wisely with a proper return on investment.

Low-Frequency Checklist/Scoring

Yes	No	Question
		Do I feel drained/tired/depleted?
		Do I feel down or depressed?
		Am I left feeling frustrated, angry, or a little hostile?
		Do I find myself immediately reaching for something to make me feel better?
		Do I feel like I need to tell someone to get guidance/feel better/validation?

Yes = 1 point

No = 0 points

Give yourself a score:

0 points: Engaging in this does not have a low-frequency effect on me.

1–2 points: Engaging in this is somewhat low frequency.

3 points: This is having a low-frequency effect on me.

4–5 points: This is having an extremely low-frequency effect and is unhealthy for me on various levels.

High-Frequency Checklist/Scoring

Yes	No	Question
		Do I feel energized and inspired?
		Do I feel happy?
		Do I feel centered and content?
		Do I feel more empowered?
		Do I feel more positive and determined?

Yes = 1 point

No = 0 points

Give yourself a score:

0 points: Engaging in this does not have a high-frequency effect on me.

1–2 points: Engaging in this is somewhat high frequency.

3 points: This is having a significant high-frequency effect on me.

4–5 points: This is having an extremely high-frequency effect and is healthy for me on various levels.

Look at your written answers and compare the two scores. You will know clearly, definitively, and quantifiably what gives you the greatest return on your attention investment and what you need to remove or add to in your life immediately.

Summary

In this chapter we learned that your most precious resource—your energy—must be used wisely and mindfully. We use energy for everything. Every thought, emotion, action, and behavior is created by the manipulation of our energy. It only stands to reason that to have the greatest, happiest, and most successful life possible, learning to master the use of your energy is paramount. It dictates everything.

We also discovered in this chapter the revolutionary energy diagnostic system. This new understanding gives you a quantifiable, repeatable, and robust tool to measure the return on investment of your energetic investments. We no longer will have to wonder which people, activities, or circumstances bring a positive return to your energy bank account or leave you depleted.

With your new understanding of how you use energy for everything, coupled with the revolutionary energy diagnostic system, you are truly empowered with the tools you need to create the life you truly desire. You now know how to measure and eliminate that which depletes your energy as well as focus on and increase what revitalizes, inspires, and increases your energy.

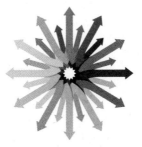

Chapter 9

Energy Diagnostics for Activities

Now that you know how the energetic diagnostic systems works and how to manage your energy bank account, it's time for you to discover what activities empower and raise your frequency and what activities disempower and drop your frequency. Measuring your return on investment is the key to success.

Here is a list of examples of activities for you to use as a template. Your checklist needs to be an accurate snapshot of your next seven days based upon your daily habits or what you "pay attention" (give energy) to.

- Exercising
- Being outdoors
- Shopping
- Looking up or researching information
- Scrolling social media
- Selecting and preparing food
- Texting/talking
- Gaming
- Binge-watching videos/movies/TV/sports
- Fantasizing about or engaging in sex/masturbation

- Fixing or adjusting your appearance
- Caring for a child or animal (companion entity)
- Engaging in a creative endeavor (writing, painting, etc.)
- Building something

Change Your Mind:
Energy Diagnostics for Activities

Your seven-day challenge is to become supremely mindful and aware regarding where your energy/attention is going. This master level of energy cognizance is going to give you the ability and power to completely transform your life.

Devote yourself completely to your energy diagnostics and the reward will be the conscious return of what you truly are: a limitless creator being capable of Self-mastery.

What You Need

Get your energy diagnostics notebook out and make your activity list.

What It Looks Like

For each activity you perform, reflect on your energy/attention frequencies. The answers to these questions need not be short stories. Simply accurately and honestly write the truth to each question.

Before

- How do I feel emotionally leading up to the activity?
- What is my thought process that proceeds the activity?
- How do I feel energetically leading up to the activity?
- How do I feel physically before I engage in the activity?

During

- How do I feel emotionally during the activity?
- What is my thought process during the activity?
- How do I feel energetically while engaged in the activity?
- How do I feel physically while engaged in the activity?

After

- How do I feel emotionally after the activity?
- What is my thought process after the activity?
- How do I feel energetically after the activity?
- How do I feel physically immediately after the activity has ended?

Now there is enough introspection and subsequent clarity regarding your state of being as it relates to your activities in order to accurately tabulate the effect they have had on your energy bank account.

Low-Frequency Checklist/Scoring

Yes	No	Question
		Do I feel drained/tired/depleted?
		Do I feel down or depressed?
		Am I left feeling frustrated, angry, or a little hostile?
		Do I find myself immediately reaching for something to make me feel better?
		Do I feel like I need to tell someone to get guidance/feel better/validation?

Yes = 1 point
No = 0 points

Give yourself a score:

0 points: Engaging in this activity does not have a low-frequency effect on me.

1–2 points: Engaging in this activity is somewhat low frequency.

3 points: This activity is having a significant low-frequency effect on me.

4–5 points: This activity is having an extremely low-frequency effect and is unhealthy for me on various levels.

High-Frequency Checklist/Scoring

Yes	No	Question
		Do I feel energized and inspired?
		Do I feel happy?
		Do I feel centered and content?
		Do I feel more empowered?
		Do I feel more determined?

Yes = 1 point

No = 0 points

Give yourself a score:

0 points: Engaging in this activity does not have a high-frequency effect on me.

1–2 points: Engaging in this activity is somewhat high frequency.

3 points: This activity is having a significant high-frequency effect on me.

4–5 points: This activity is having an extremely high-frequency effect on me and is healthy on various levels.

Look at your written answers and compare the two scores. You will know definitively and quantifiably what gives you the greatest return on your attention investment and what you need to increase/remove from your life immediately.

Client Examples

Several of my clients underwent the twenty-one-day challenge with the last seven days being dedicated to their energy diagnostics. I am sharing their experiences here as examples of what they did and how it worked for them—as it will for you. I omitted their fourteen-day notebook challenge work as it does not directly correlate to this specific section.

Rebecca

Rebecca is an intelligent, sincere, and compassionate young woman in her late twenties. She lives on the Big Island of Hawaii and is studying to become an energy healer and intuitive reader. After taking an advanced healing course with me, she has transcended the traumatic emotional and mental baggage from growing up in a severely dysfunctional family and, in doing so, overcame an extremely debilitating three-year case of Lyme disease.

Now that she has overcome her myriad health issues over the last year and feels much better physically, she has found herself really struggling with all the problems she sees in the world. She feels defeated by all the constant low-frequency turmoil, manipulation, negativity, and division. She scheduled a session with me in the hopes of getting out of the downward spiral she was in.

"RJ, I can't shake this sense of utter hopelessness. I am doing everything I can to be healthier and more aware and awake, but the world is such a mess. I feel like there is no point."

"No point in what?"

"In trying to wake people up. The more I investigate things, the more horrified I am. Everything I believed in was a lie. It's overwhelming. How could I have been so fooled by it all? It gets worse by the day, and I don't want to participate in this world."

Rebecca, like roughly 40 percent of the world population from my perspective, has been on an awakening and healing journey these last several years. And like many who seek tangible truth, in all its forms, she has been shaken to her core.

"Rebecca, in the low frequencies of the physical universe, where you and I are right now, deception, coercion, and corruption is inherent. That's what our subconscious, patterned, egoic mind is built upon and belongs to. We can all very easily succumb to the lower frequencies, and many of us do."

"Why?"

"Because our physical environment and world culture are extremely low frequency. It's like falling asleep. Before you realize it, you're unconscious. It's easy to fool people when they are already fooling themselves. They are disconnected, consciously, from their true essence. Hence, people give up on themselves and each other because it's easy. People go along with what they are told because it's easy. This is all part of what makes being here so challenging."

Rebecca nodded in agreement as she jotted down a quick note in her journal.

"Rebecca, let's look at how you are spending your most precious resource, your attention. Attention is energy. Where your attention goes, your energy flows. It's possible you need to reevaluate your return on investment, meaning what you are paying attention to and what your energetic takeaway is."

"I never thought of energy and attention as the same thing, but it makes perfect sense. Yes, let's look. What do I need to do?"

I advised her to take stock of what she is paying attention to during her normal day. I explained the very simple questions she must ask herself prior, during, and after her activities. That would give her a much clearer understanding of the energetic cost regarding her most precious resource and what her return on investment was.

I then shared with her the simple energetic diagnostic scoring system and how to tally her results, giving her a quantifiable metric that she can use for all her activities. She agreed to put the system in place, and we would go over the results during our session next week.

One week later, it was obvious the moment Rebecca came up on screen that she was feeling better. Her smile was ear to ear and her increased energy level was palpable.

"Is this the same Rebecca I spoke with last week?" I joked.

She laughed and flipped open her journal.

"Not even close. I feel so much better. This was incredible, RJ."

"Do tell."

"By using the energy diagnostic system, I finally took stock of what I was paying attention to. You were right. I had some terrible investments. The biggest one was all the constant research I was doing on all the things the media never addresses or totally fabricates and spins."

"What did you learn?"

"I learned that even though much of what I suspected was true, unfortunately, I realized the whole process was making me feel depressed, angry, and hopeless. It wasn't improving my quality of life; it was robbing me off it."

"There's a law of diminishing returns here. Once you know, move on. Otherwise, it becomes draining and disempowering."

"Very. When I measured this specific activity—all the researching I was doing—I got a very high score on the disempowering/ low-frequency energy diagnostics. I was depleting my energy bank account big time. I also realized how much it was negatively affecting me in several other facets of my life."

"Can you give me an example?"

"I would feel contempt for all the people who didn't know what I knew. It made me angry and depressed. In turn, I would isolate myself out of frustration. This led to indulging in other activities that resulted in a poor return on investment, like binge-watching TV or scrolling social media.

"These are fantastic insights, Rebecca."

"It's totally life altering. I see that I was not living the way I wanted or was capable of. One bad energy investment had snowballed into so many facets of my life I had no idea until now."

"You are clearly happier, more energetic, and wiser for putting in the effort."

"Thanks, RJ. Now I have an easy system that keeps me operating at a much higher energy level, and it gives me awesome insight into my attention-based return on investment."

Rebecca now has a great understanding of the highest use of her most sacred gift: her attention. She has cut out over-researching, binge-watching, and scrolling through social media. She now feels infinitely happier, more positive, and empowered.

Jeremiah

Jeremiah is in his late twenties and lives in Los Angeles, California. He lives at home with his parents and is currently unemployed. He graduated from college about six years ago and worked steadily until the pandemic. He was let go about year and a half ago and has not been able to find work since.

Jeremiah read my first book, *Supercharged Self-Healing*, after watching a few interviews I did on YouTube. He then booked a session with me through my website. In his email, he said he needed help getting out of the rut he found himself in. He stated that he has tried everything, but nothing seems to work or stick for very long. I logged on to our scheduled virtual meeting right on time. Jeremiah was already waiting for me.

"Nice to meet you, Jeremiah."

"I'm really excited to speak with you, RJ."

"Likewise. I read the notes you sent. Why don't you tell me what's going on, and we can go from there."

"Okay. I guess the best way to say it is that I feel like I've lost all joy and motivation in my life. I can't find a job. I live at home with my parents. I don't have a girlfriend. I feel like I'm stuck, and I don't know how to turn things around."

"I understand. What do you want your life to be?"

Jeremiah paused. He was truly contemplating the question I just posed to him.

"I want to have something I'm excited about doing. I don't want to live at home anymore. I want someone in my life—a girlfriend. I feel like I have no life."

His loneliness, frustration, and Self-loathing were palpable. I intuited a deep resentment for how he sees the world. I knew where we needed to go.

"Jeremiah, for me to help you as much as I can, I need you to be brutally honest with yourself and with me. Can you do that?"

This was the moment of truth for Jeremiah, and he knew it. He blinked a few times, took a deep breath, and nodded his head in agreement.

"Yes."

"Great. Now we can get somewhere, my friend. How do you spend your day, Jeremiah? Be honest and be specific."

Jeremiah swallowed hard. He was summoning the courage to look in the mirror and speak the truth. I was already proud of him.

"I get high as soon as I wake up. I, uh…"

Jeremiah broke his gaze with me and looked down. He needed to pause before he could admit more. I held the space for him.

"After I get high, I watch porn and masturbate. I just kind of do that every day before I get out of bed."

I nodded silently to acknowledge his admission and for him for to continue.

"Then I scroll through social media for a while. Just mindlessly, really. I'm not looking for anything. I look through the news feed that comes through. It's just more constant horrifying stuff. It's all fear and lies."

He returned his gaze to me, and I met him with total nonjudgment. I nodded as I wanted him to feel comfortable and continue.

"I'll scroll through Tinder for a while, but it's pointless. I don't feel good enough about myself to contact anybody. I don't even know why I look anymore."

His frustration, anger, and despair were starting to come to the surface.

"Every job that comes through my feed is for some soulless corporation. It's all phony virtue signaling. I can't do it. It's all totally empty. I'm not motivated by money. I would rather be homeless than sell my soul. There is nothing here for me anymore. There's nothing."

With his truthful admission, Jeremiah no longer had to hide anymore. It was all out in the open now. He did not have to suffer the intensity of his frustration, hopelessness, anger, and despair alone.

"Jeremiah, thank you for being so honest. And for the courage it took to share intimate details about how you feel."

I could tell Jeremiah was getting emotional. He was staring blankly at his computer keyboard. His eyes were watering, and his breathing was getting shorter. I needed to acknowledge this and let him know that I am here for him.

"Look at me," I commanded with great power. His watery eyes met mine, and I locked into his. I emanated my full presence and poured my power and love right into him. "I promise you will never have to suffer these things again. From this moment on, you shall never carry this pain within your heart. Those days are over. You are free of your suffering. Do you hear me, Jeremiah?"

Jeremiah completely broke. He wept uncontrollably. The tears streamed down his cheeks, and his shoulders shuddered from the force. I remained as I AM. The pain and hurt he released was profound. I said nothing as words were no longer needed. Eventually, he began to calm down.

"From now on, you shall talk to yourself the way you'd talk to someone you love. You will be warm, compassionate, and forgiving toward yourself even when you struggle, feel not good enough, or even fail."

"I am not sure I know how to do that, RJ."

"I will show you. The activities and habits you're giving your attention to are robbing you of your energy and your will. These things are not empowering you and raising your frequency. On the contrary, they are profoundly disempowering you and dropping your frequency. It's why you no longer feel good about yourself or have the sufficient energy to make wholesale changes."

"I feel that—big time."

"There is no way we can create the life we want if we are paying attention to everything other than what we want to manifest. Attention is energy, and you must give your attention to precisely what you want to grow."

"I totally get it. After you say it, it seems so obvious…and simple."

"The truth is simple. The death of the subconscious, patterned, egoic mind is the birth of wisdom."

I instructed Jeremiah on how to begin the energy diagnostic system. He needed to see the return on investment on what he was giving his attention/energy to. Once you see it—tangibly, quantifiably—it gives you permission and motivation to transform yourself and your life. Jeremiah was all in. We agreed to reconvene in a few weeks and go from there.

I must admit, I logged in to Jeremiah about ten days after our session. When I "log in" someone or something, I use higher-intuitive functions like clairsentience, clairvoyance, or claircognizance (among others) to read the energies associated with the person or thing. It gives me a far more holistic and clearer understanding of what is going on energetically on myriad levels.

Based upon what I perceived, I knew our session three weeks later was going to be very different from our initial meeting. Once the day came, I didn't have to wait long because Jeremiah, just like with our first session, was already waiting and ready to go. When Jeremiah popped up on screen, he was beaming.

"Well, look at you."

It must have been contagious because a huge smile spread across my face too.

"RJ, I don't know if I have ever felt like this in my life. I did exactly what you instructed. The very first thing I did was, I would take a minute and write down how I was feeling before I engaged in any of my daily activities. I looked at my thoughts, how I was feeling, even physically before I would do anything."

"Perfect."

"I stayed totally mindful about what my state of being was while engaged in the habits and activities. I would even stop and write down exactly what was going on with me mentally, emotionally, and physically while in the middle of it. Just doing that I cannot believe how much I learned. My mind is blown."

"This is true Self-awareness, Jeremiah. Keep going; this is so wonderful to hear."

"Then I would do the same thing after the activity ended. It was just a few sentences, but I really took stock of how I felt after. Then I ran the energy diagnostics on my activities and tallied my score."

"What did you learn, tangibly and quantifiably, after writing and calculating your score?"

"I learned more about myself and why I was doing these things and what I was not doing in the last three weeks than I could have ever imagined. This is what needs to be taught in freakin' schools. It's mind-boggling. I now know about subconscious programming and how attention and energy really work. It dictates your entire life."

"Spoken like a true wizard, my friend."

"Pretty much everything I was doing was having a disempowering and low-frequency effect on me. I was giving all my energy to stuff that didn't give me what I wanted. Now I know why I was doing it. I felt worse and respected myself less after. I was depleting my energy bank account all day, every day. It was so obvious why I felt so hopeless and depressed with myself and my life."

"The first step in alchemical transformation is to recognize our return on investment in regard to our attention—our energy."

"I get it now. Once I saw it—the words, my scores—it made it easy. It totally hit home. I have cut out all my poor energetic investments. All of them. I feel 1,000 percent better. I'm finally capable and ready to create the life I want for myself. I know what to do now. I am so grateful. Thank you, RJ."

"No need to thank me. You did all the work. I knew you would."

Jeremiah finally feels free of the hopelessness, despair, Self-loathing, and frustration he had felt and been carrying around the last several years. He understands one of the essential keys to transformation: where your attention goes, your energy flows.

Summary

Being acutely mindful of the activities you perform gives you immense power. Knowing how you are spending your energy and what the return on investment is changes your life. From a metaphysical perspective, what you do with your energy is your life. In other words, your discipline is your destiny. With your new ninja-level awareness of your activities, you are now operating with formidable power and true clarity.

Investigate new activities as you remove poor performing ones. Let your increased clarity regarding yourself be your guide. Often, after deleting an old activity and choosing a new activity, any activity (within reason) is often better than stagnation. With your energy diagnostic system, you will quickly, accurately, and quantifiably measure the return on investment regarding your new activity. There is no need to be hesitant if you feel like stagnation may be setting in. You have the tools you need. Go for it.

Activities that are worth spending your energy expenditure on are those that uplift you, center you, empower you, and liberate you. Be ruthlessly mindful about your activities. They truly dictate the quality of your life. Being ferocious about protecting and enhancing your energetic integrity through the activities you engage in, or don't engage in, is a sign that portends greatness. Do not be afraid to be powerful, clear, and definitive with your activities while always maintaining an open mind. Oddly enough, you will find, along with your increased focus and power, that there is a gentleness and tenderness in how you treat yourself and others.

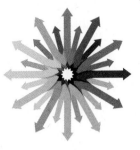

Chapter 10

Energy Diagnostics
for Personal Relationships

The voice inside your head (Self-talk) dictates your moment-to-moment existence. That voice is your programming, not the Real You. All your behavior is dictated by your subconscious, patterned, egoic mind. The work you are doing now by utilizing this book is essential in your ability to change your mind and, subsequently, change your life.

The company you keep (besides the voice in your head) also has a massive effect on you and the quality of your life. Many—if not all—of your beliefs have been dictated to you by what you have put your attention upon. Being able to tangibly see and quantifiably measure the return on investment regarding whom you have in your life will be revelatory and beyond profound.

After doing your interpersonal energy diagnostics, you may be surprised at your results. If someone (or a few people) ends up having a greater low-frequency effect on you, rather than a high-frequency effect, it doesn't necessarily mean that you should completely cut them out of your life. Instead, it may mean that you need to take a moment to reevaluate the energy exchange going on.

If you find that all or many of the people in your life are having a low-frequency effect on you, it may be a good idea to examine why you feel this way. Examining what beliefs/expectations you have about how others should be/do/act—as well as the beliefs/expectations you have about yourself regarding relationships—will prove illuminating and extraordinarily beneficial.

Change Your Mind:
Energy Diagnostics for Interpersonal Relationships

Just as you ran energy diagnostics on your attention/energy and activities, you can run diagnostics on the people you interact with. Use your energy notebook and answer the questions below for each person you interact with on a deeper level. Here is a quick review on how to commence with your energy diagnostics for interpersonal relationships.

Before you engage:

- How do I feel emotionally leading up to interacting with this person?
- What is my thought process that proceeds my interaction with this person?
- How do I feel energetically leading up to interacting with this person?
- How do I feel physically before I interact with this person?

During engagement:

- How do I feel emotionally while interacting with this person?
- What is my thought process during the interaction with this person?
- How do I feel energetically while interacting with this person?
- How do I feel physically while interacting with this person?

After engagement:

- How do I feel emotionally after the interaction with this person?
- What is my thought process after the interaction with this person?
- How do I feel energetically after interacting with this person?
- How do I feel physically immediately after interacting with this person?

Remember, the answers to these questions do not need to be verbose or long-winded. The more concise you can be with your answers, the clearer you are regarding your state of being. Once you have completed the written part of your energy diagnostics, move on to tabulating your energy bank account score.

Low-Frequency Checklist/Scoring

Yes	No	Question
		Do I feel drained/tired/depleted?
		Do I feel down or depressed?
		Am I left feeling frustrated, angry, or a little hostile?
		Do I find myself immediately reaching for something to make me feel better?
		Do I feel like I need to tell someone about them to get guidance/feel better/validation?

Yes = 1 point
No = 0 points

Give yourself a score:

0 points: Engaging with this person does not have a low-frequency effect on me.

1–2 points: Engaging with this person is somewhat low frequency.

3 points: This person is having a low-frequency effect on me.

4–5 points: This person is having an extremely low-frequency effect on me and is unhealthy on various levels.

High-Frequency Checklist/Scoring

Yes	No	Question
		Do I feel energized and inspired?
		Do I feel happy?
		Do I feel centered and content?
		Do I feel more empowered?
		Do I feel more determined?

Yes = 1 point

No = 0 points

Give yourself a score:

0 points: Engaging with this person does not have a high-frequency effect on me.

1–2 points: Engaging with this person is somewhat high frequency.

3 points: This person is having a high-frequency effect on me.

4–5 points: This person is having an extremely high-frequency effect on me and is healthy on various levels.

Look at your written answers and compare the two scores. You will know definitively and quantifiably what gives you the greatest return on investment of your attention and what relationships you need to reevaluate, eliminate, or foster.

Client Examples

Several of my clients underwent the twenty-one-day challenge with the last seven days being dedicated to their energy diagnostics. I am sharing their experiences here as examples of what they did and how it worked for them—as it will for you. I omitted their fourteen-day

notebook challenge work as it does not directly correlate to this specific section.

Candice

Candice is in her mid-forties, married, and lives in Seattle, Wash-
ington. She is a data engineer for a huge multinational corporation.
Exceedingly intelligent, shy, and intensely private, she is an acquain-
tance of a client of mine. In her email to me, she said that after much
consideration and equal parts consternation, she decided to book a
session with me.

Ninety-nine times out of one hundred, I do not have the time or
bandwidth to "log in" to a new client prior to our session. I enjoy
having my first interaction with someone new be completely fresh,
so to speak. Information can—and does—often pour in simply by
reading someone's email. For some reason, I consciously kept the
flow of energetic information at a distance as I read Candice's email.

It was time to get to work. I took a sip of my hazelnut double
espresso and opened the VPN browser on my laptop. I logged in to
my Zoom account, clicked on the first of the day's scheduled client
meetings, and Candice popped right up on screen.

"Hi, Candice. Very nice to meet you."

"Very nice to meet you as well, RJ. It's so weird that I am talking
with you after reading your book and seeing so many of your interviews."

"Candice, I'm really questioning your intelligence that—after all
that forewarning—you still want to speak with me."

She laughed. I could tell she was anxious and perhaps a bit intim-
idated. A good laugh puts the nerves at ease.

"I'm glad you did, though. What is it that you would like to address
today?"

Candice adjusted her glasses and cleared her throat. "I feel like I
am closed off with people. Even with my husband, and we have a great
relationship. I'm just not comfortable around people anymore. My
friends, too. Maybe it's because of all the isolation from the pandemic,

but now that I am around people again, it's only gotten worse. I don't know what is happening with me."

I already intuitively knew what Candice needed to see and understand. Without hesitation, I got right to the heart of the matter. "What are you protecting?"

This question hit Candice like an unexpected splash of water to the face. She sat back in her chair and blinked her eyes, searching for an answer.

"I'm not sure. I just know that I don't want anyone to know what I think or how I really feel about things."

"You don't want anyone to know or just those close to you?"

Candice's eyes got wider. For her to come to certain realizations about her thought patterns, feelings, and behaviors, the curtain shielding her subconscious, egoic world needed to be torn down. For those with strong intellects, this can often be daunting, frightening, and even embarrassing.

"It's worse if they are close to me. Far worse."

Now we were getting somewhere.

"Why?"

"Because I'm far more vulnerable with people who are close to me. They could really hurt me."

"Hurt what, exactly? Forget feelings for a moment. Hurt what?"

Candice sat back. She searched the depths of her mind for an answer. She was about to break new ground regarding this problem if she was honest and courageous.

"My sense of me. Who I am as a person."

"Can someone hurt your inner sense of Self? Is that even possible? Aren't you the only one that determines that?"

Candice thought long and hard, but I could tell she needed help to dig deeper.

"I have an idea, Candice. I am going to share with you a very simple yet incredibly powerful way to uncover, resolve, and move past this problem. Does that sound good?"

"Yes. Very much. I want to understand what is going on with me. I'm not afraid to look in the mirror anymore."

That was all I needed to hear. I explained the notebook exercise and energy diagnostic system to Candice. She was more than interested and took copious notes. It was obvious that she was fiercely determined to get to the core of her lifelong problem and defeat it once and for all. We agreed to speak again in a few weeks to unpack her new discoveries.

Three weeks later, I was interested to see what Candice discovered since our initial meeting. There is a very interesting phenomenon that takes place during sessions with clients. I realized a very long time ago that what I may tangibly and unequivocally understand/see/know about someone doesn't matter. It's only what they tangibly realize about themselves that carries the real power of alchemical transformation.

On the deepest levels, it makes no difference that I could see what Candice could not. What does matter is that the precise nectar and elixir is brewed for the blossoming of Self-awareness. This flowering provides the intoxicating perfume of gnosis that sweetly fills your every breath. This is the only directive, the only truth, the only mandate of existence; know thyself.

It was time for my session with Candice. Whatever it was that she discovered about herself was a step in the right direction. I was ready for my session. All I needed at this point was my day planner and for my laptop to be as charged as I was from my vanilla-flavored double espresso!

"Hi, Candice. Nice to see you.

"Nice to see you too."

"How have you been since we last spoke?"

"Incredible. Absolutely incredible."

"Sounds positively intriguing. Do tell."

"By doing the energy diagnostics, which is truly amazing by the way, I discovered a significantly poor return on investment with my mom. It was so bad that it affected pretty much all the returns on my interpersonal relationships. I always knew there was a real problem with our relationship, but now I see it clearly."

"What did you discover specifically?"

"I was always shy and protective of myself. As an adult, I have become a bit of a recluse. Now I know why. I was protecting myself from my mom. She has a way that makes me feel completely invalidated. My perspective and my feelings were simply wrong. At an early age, I must have decided the best way to operate was to never reveal my inner life for fear of being discounted."

"What brought this to light recently?"

"My husband and I went to my parents' for my dad's seventy-sixth birthday. I asked myself the questions about what I was thinking, feeling, and how I was doing physically before we left. It was so revealing and undeniable now that I saw the words right in front of my eyes. I did the quick energy diagnostics before, during, and after the birthday dinner. The return on investment was off-the-charts negative."

"How do you feel now, seeing and knowing, quantifiably, how you are impacted by your interactions with your mom?"

"My first reaction was that I was never going to speak with her again. It's that bad. I've been denying it my whole life, but now I can't anymore. But I thought about it, and what I really want is to change the energy exchange, not end the relationship. So, the next weekend I went back to my parents' house. I brought all my notes and scores and showed my mom just how our relationship affects me."

"How did she take it?"

"At first, all she did was defend herself and project everything onto me. I told her she doesn't even need to say anything but to please try and see there is more to our relationship than just her perspective of it. And that I have been hurt by it, and I want and need it to be better. Otherwise, I am not going to keep participating in something that continually hurts me to my core."

"I'm proud of you. How did you two leave it?"

"Surprisingly, she is open to change. Maybe me thinking she won't be open to this was just a projection of mine. In fact, she said she wants to do the energy diagnostics too! Once she saw what I wrote and the scores, it really made her step back."

"That's fantastic."

"It is. I also discovered how protecting myself from my mom developed into a personality trait, my ego mind. It affects every relationship I have, including the one I have with myself. By seeing the return on investment with my mom, I can address improving all the interpersonal relationships I have. I already feel more relaxed and less on guard around people."

"There is nothing to really protect, is there?"

"No, now that I see why I felt that way, it's gone. It no longer dictates my behavior. My entire thought process has radically changed. How I feel and act has radically changed too. It's astonishing."

Candice has changed her life by consciously seeing and tangibly understanding what is driving her behavior and affecting her energy. You have the same ability to change your life as well. Only by bringing the patterned, subconscious, egoic mind into full view do we realize we have the power to transcend all programmed limitations.

Sara

Sara is in her early thirties and lives in Tarpon Springs, Florida. She is a divorced stay-at-home mother of three young children. She lives in her stepfather's house and is his caretaker. She also volunteers at a local food shelter every Saturday and is an avid swimmer. She suffers from anxiety, chronic fatigue, migraines, depression, poor digestive health, and insomnia.

I treated her sister, who lives in San Diego. Her sister, Christine, had been diagnosed with bipolar disorder, depression, and night terrors. Based upon the success Christine had, along with encouragement from her, Sara decided to book a remote video session with me.

In Sara's email to me, I sensed what the root cause of her struggles were. In fact, Sara's symptoms are quite common for a lot of people. She said, in her introductory email, that all her ailments began with the birth of her first child, Jack, roughly thirteen years ago. They have gotten increasingly worse since the birth of her two other children. She has had no success with the Western medicine pharmaceutical paradigm and only limited success with alternative therapies.

I sat down in my chair, flipped open my laptop, and clicked into my virtual meetings.

"Hi, Sara. Nice to meet you."

"Nice to meet you too. My sister, Christine, can't stop raving about you. I always knew it was a matter of time before I reached out."

"I'm glad you did. How can I help?"

"I am a mess. Everything affects me. Everything. My anxiety is off the charts. I don't sleep well, so I'm totally exhausted all the time. I can't think straight because I'm so sleep deprived. My stomach is always upset. I can't really eat anything."

"I understand."

"I feel like I never have a moment to myself. Between the kids and my stressed-out stepfather, I just feel totally overwhelmed. He's old and has been sick. He expects me to take care of him, take him to his appointments, talk to all the specialists, oversee his health care, and literally manage his entire life. It's just too much."

"Taking care of ill family members can be extremely stressful, on top of everything else we have on our plate."

"It's more than that. I don't even know who I am anymore. All the stuff that I have made to be so important in my life feels completely empty and meaningless. We have a nice house, cars, and money from my divorce, but we're all miserable. Everybody is constantly sick and stressed out. It's like my life is managing stuff, scheduling things, cleaning up after people, making sure everybody is okay. It all falls on me. I'm overwhelmed and depressed. It's like I have no joy in my life."

Sara broke down. As she sobbed, her hands shook in her attempt to wipe away the torrent of tears. Her frail shoulders, which poked through her soft, blue cashmere sweater, bobbed up and down from the surge of emotions. She tried to regain her composure, but the intensity of her feelings was too much.

"It's okay, Sara. Let it out. It's okay."

I held the space for her. A space nobody gives her, and one she doesn't know how to give herself—yet. There was no need to speak because my vibrational broadcast spoke in a fullness that words cannot.

"How long did I last without crying? Two minutes?"

"That's waaaay longer than a lot of people I talk to; trust me."

She laughed.

"Sara, listen to me. There is nothing wrong with you. Absolutely nothing. None of these symptoms belong to you. You need to understand this."

This stopped Sara in her tracks. Her crying immediately ceased, and the huge emotional waves completely flatlined like a placid body of water. Not a ripple in sight.

"What do you mean?"

"You are an empath. Do you know what that is?"

"No, not really. I've heard the term before, but I'm not familiar with what it means."

"Empaths are extraordinarily sensitive Souls. Everything affects them. An empath picks up on other people's emotions and thoughts and is massively impacted by them. It's so overwhelming, empaths can't differentiate their own thoughts, feelings, and stressors from those that belong to others. It's way too much to process."

"That is exactly how I feel."

"You lose your own sense of Self because of the constant mental and emotional contagion from others. You don't know what's you anymore. Your stress and anxiety, your insomnia, your digestive issues, your lack of joy—it's because you are an empath."

"Is this normal?"

"For you, it is. My understanding is that roughly 5 percent of the population is sensitive with about 1 percent being truly empathic. And you are truly empathic."

"This is like a curse."

"Empaths are on this planet to alchemize all the low-frequency thoughts and emotions of the planet. More evolved Souls do this as a way of healing everyone. You're a healer; all empaths are. You just don't realize it or know how to work with your sensitivity properly."

Sara's entire world completely shifted in one instant. This hit Sara so hard. She just stared at me wide-eyed and speechless. Her mind was connecting all the dots in her life experiences. She finally got the hidden truth to all her lifelong unanswerable questions and chronic ill health.

"This is incredible. It makes perfect sense. Now I know why nothing has ever really worked for me. Western pharmaceuticals, Eastern medicine. Medications, tinctures, herbs, meditation, sound bowl therapy, even shamanic journeying. Nothing has ever been more than just a temporary fix."

"Those things will never work because being an empath is an aspect of the Self—what you really are. It isn't to be treated or drugged; it's a talent and ability that is part of your very essence."

"What should I do?"

"The first thing I suggest is the deprogramming of your subconscious, patterned, egoic mind. You must see how all your energetic indentations and identifications do not belong to you. That is the only place to ever start."

"How do I do that?"

"I'm going to show you how to bring the subconscious mind into your conscious awareness and understanding. After you do this, you will run simple but powerful energy diagnostics. This will show you who is affecting your energy the most. You must become aware of what you are paying attention to and what the effect is. You are going to learn things about yourself you can't even imagine right now. You are going to be able to turn all of this around."

"Sounds great but really daunting."

"Be prepared to see yourself, your life, your relationships, and the world with far greater clarity."

"RJ, I'm so ready. I am exhausted, stressed, sick, depressed, and have gotten so far away from having any real joy in my life. I am willing to do anything to be healthy and happy."

"Then let's get to it."

I explained to Sara both the notebook exercise and the energy diagnostic system. I emphasized to her that it is only upon bringing the subconscious, patterned, egoic mind into the awareness of the conscious mind that you can affect real transformation, and not mere change because change implies a residue of the past. Transformation speaks to your natural abilities as a limitless creator being.

As you do the work outlined in this book, realize you are not merely thinking outside the box—you are removing the box. This is the key to the transcendence of agreed-upon human limitations. There is no block or resistance to anything. Your only bondage is not realizing this.

I was particularly interested to see how Sara had been doing during her three weeks of diagnostics. She really did give herself quite a challenge being a true empath. It's hard enough to shed the subconscious, patterned, egoic mind, but doing so while receiving a constant flow of low-frequency disharmonious energies forces you to raise your game by an order of magnitude.

Sara is not only an empath, but she is also raising three young kids on her own. She also has several companion entities as well. Two dogs, three cats, and one bird, to be exact. I absolutely love animals as well. They remind us of what unconditional love is. I have a feeling it's Sara's companion entities that, without her even realizing it, have helped keep her sane through their love.

There was something else I picked up when speaking with Sara. And this, too, was something that did not belong to her. I opened my day planner, turned on my computer, and took a hearty sip of my delicious homemade Mexican mocha coffee with two shots of espresso and extra whip. It tastes better than it sounds (if that's even possible).

"Hola, chica! Nice to see you, Sara!"

"Nice to see you again, too, RJ. I've been really looking forward to this."

"And why is that?"

"These teachings are so life changing and eye-opening, I can't believe it."

"That's what I like to hear. Tell me what the last few weeks have been like for you and what you've discovered."

"Where do I start?! First, I did the notebook exercise. Do people know that everything they do is because of their programming and egoic identity? I am still in total disbelief at how deep this stuff is ingrained into our psyche. I can't believe how much better I feel, how much lighter I feel since doing it. It's like all the problems of the world have left me."

"All problems need your approval to exist."

"Fascinating. This was the first time in my entire life that I really took stock of what I was doing, feeling, thinking, and why. It's the why. I could see all of my constant motion and seeking. It was never-ending and exhausting. No wonder I was totally exhausted just from that."

"To seek is to stress; to align is to rest."

A huge smile broke out across Sara's face. "Now I really understand that statement. It would never have been doable until now."

Her smile was contagious. I nodded and Sara continued, "It was my need to be in control of everything, to make everything fit the conditioning of my patterned, subconscious mind and egoic identity. I have been so afraid to let life happen and therefore enjoy it because I have been trying to live up to my false identity by controlling life. It's because I was so controlled! It was all driven by fear of not being able to be the perfect daughter, wife, and mom. I have suffered my entire life because of that fear. My mind was always going and going and now I really understand why. Fear. And a lack of Self-awareness."

"The most persistent and detrimental suffering is the addiction to identity."

"My God, you're so right. I have never even met myself, my True Self, until now. I can't believe it. And once you see all the programming, right there on paper in front of your face, it's like it immediately loses its power. It leaves you, finally."

"Exactly. The key is to shine a light on the hidden puppeteer, the subconscious, patterned, egoic mind."

"This is the best thing I have ever done for myself, ever. I can't thank you enough."

"There is nothing to thank me for. You did all the work, Sara. You did it."

"Thanks, RJ."

"Tell me about the energy diagnostics you did."

"Holy cow. You are so right about what I was paying attention to. It was leaving me disempowered, stressed, nervous, and exhausted. My return on investment was horrifying. All I was doing was depleting my energy repeatedly to control everything."

"What was the worst return in regard to your attention?"

"My stepfather. I focused so much on his stress, his wants, his demands, his outlook, his brainwashed mind, his need to have things a certain way, that I had nothing for me. Nothing. I could never actually be myself."

This was what I picked up regarding Sara earlier. Her being an empath and being connected and always around someone who operates in a low-frequency way was extremely detrimental to Sara. Extremely.

"I had no idea why I had so much trouble sleeping until now. I was picking all of this up from him. I felt no joy in my life because most of my attention was on him and my kids, and he is always stressed out, normally sick, wanting something, and can't sit still. I can't either, and I was never like this. It's him. He is my worst return on investment."

"How do you feel about that?"

"Now that I know it's not me, I already feel much better. We are all going on a mini-vacation, and I can't wait to share all this with him. I want him and I to be on the same page. I need for us to be on the same page. I'm too sensitive. I feel like I finally have my voice back, and I'm going use it."

"I'm very proud of you, Sara. It takes courage to look in the mirror, do the work, and live truthfully."

"I have three kids, RJ, and I'm not getting any younger. I owe it to them. They need the best version of myself. They need it, and so do I."

Sara is a different person from just three weeks ago. She is finally herself for the first time in her entire life. She also has an understanding and a quantifiable metric of how she spends her most precious resource: her attention. These two insights might be the most valuable lessons we ever learn.

Summary

From my own higher-consciousness exploration, I discovered that a very long time ago, hundreds of millions of years ago, the very first humans lead an incredibly solitary existence. I won't get into the specifics here, but suffice it to say, the human experience, regarding its inception and conception, was not directed toward relationships with the other explorers of the "human condition." Fast-forward to today and most of our actions (all for the evolution of our consciousness) are relationship based, personal or otherwise.

Anytime you interact or even respond to anyone, you are establishing and therefore agreeing to an energy exchange. It will, most assuredly, alter your field of energy and your overall vibrational frequency. You now can be supremely confident and crystal clear in the evaluation of past, present, and future relationship choices you make. Through the repeatable, robust, and quantifiable way to measure the energetic effect of any relationship you engage in and its effect upon you, you have the right tool to build the best relationships for you.

Only the subconscious, patterned, egoic mind defines itself by things outside of itself. Most of us do this with great suffering regarding our personal relationships. The only toxic relationship we ever have is with our own programmed mind, and it plays itself out with every interpersonal relationship we ever have. All rules were meant to be broken once you've escaped the prison and tyranny of your patterned, subconscious mind. You, my friend, are no longer playing by the same rules as you did prior to reading this book. You're not even playing the same game.

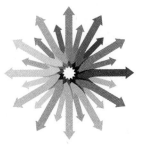

Chapter 11

Energy Diagnostics for Circumstances/Events

Many of us live our lives in a very familiar, habitual, and predictable way. Rarely, if ever, do we examine or measure what is happening, metaphysically, to our brain and energy when we engage is these habitual circumstances/events. Even more rare is to quantifiably compare these habits against one another.

This energetic diagnostic is essential to discover what circumstances/events raise your frequency and empower you and which ones drop your frequency and disempower you. As you now well know, your most precious resource is attention because where your attention goes, your energy flows. It is essential you know your return on investment on what circumstances/events you are paying attention to.

Start by simply asking yourself these two sets of questions:

"Who is participating in these events?"
    Answer: "Me, I am."
    Question: "Who am I?"

"Who is putting themselves in these circumstances?"
    Answer: "Me, I am."
    Question: "Who am I?"

Take note how you feel after just asking those two simple questions. They may very well illuminate who/what is driving your behavior. Often, the who and what are both the same illusion: your patterned, subconscious, egoic mind. Try it and see what you discover. Remember to always notebook your answers.

Change Your Mind:
Energy Diagnostics for Circumstances/Events

Use the following checklist and scoring to examine further if any of your daily or occasional events/circumstances have a high-frequency/empowering or low-frequency/disempowering effect on you.

Here are a few examples of events/circumstances for your energy diagnostic system:

- Being at work
- Work meetings
- Holiday gatherings
- Parties
- Family dinners
- Nights out (with friends)
- Sporting events
- Concerts
- Dates
- Belonging to social groups
- Belonging to health groups
- Belonging to political groups
- Belonging to religious groups

As always, ask yourself the following questions and notebook the answers.

Before engaging:

- How do I feel emotionally leading up to this circumstance/event?

- What is my thought process that proceeds this circumstance /event?
- How do I feel energetically leading up to this circumstance/ event?
- How do I feel physically before the circumstance/event?

During engagement:

- How do I feel emotionally while experiencing this circumstance/event?
- What is my thought process during the circumstance/ event?
- How do I feel energetically during the circumstance/event?
- How do I feel physically during the circumstance/event?

After engagement:

- How do I feel emotionally after the circumstance/event?
- What is my thought process after the circumstance/event?
- How do I feel energetically after the circumstance/event?
- How do I feel physically immediately after the circumstance/event?

Low-Frequency Checklist/Scoring

Yes	No	Question
		Do I feel drained/tired/depleted?
		Do I feel down or depressed?
		Am I left feeling frustrated, angry, or a little hostile?
		Do I find myself immediately reaching for something to make me feel better?
		Do I feel like I need to tell someone to get guidance/feel better/validation?

Yes = 1 point

No = 0 points

Give yourself a score:

0 points: This circumstance/event does not have a low-frequency effect on me.

1–2 points: This circumstance/event is somewhat low frequency.

3 points: This circumstance/event is having a low-frequency effect on me.

4–5 points: This circumstance/event is having an extremely low-frequency effect on me and is unhealthy on various levels.

High-Frequency Checklist/Scoring

Yes	No	Question
		Do I feel energized and inspired?
		Do I feel happy?
		Do I feel centered and content?
		Do I feel more empowered?
		Do I feel more determined?

Yes = 1 point

No = 0 points

Give yourself a score:

0 points: Participating in this circumstance/event does not have a high-frequency effect on me.

1–2 points: Participating in this circumstance/event is somewhat high frequency.

3 points: This circumstance/event is having a significant high-frequency effect on me.

4–5 points: This circumstance/event is having an extremely high-frequency effect on me and is healthy on various levels.

Look at your written answers and compare the two scores. You will know definitively and quantifiably what gives you the greatest return on investment for your attention and what you need to remove from your life.

Client Examples

Several of my clients underwent the twenty-one-day challenge with the last seven days being dedicated to their energy diagnostics. I am sharing their experiences here as examples of what they did and how it worked for them—as it will for you. I omitted their fourteen-day notebook challenge work as it does not directly correlate to this specific section.

Carl

Carl is a very successful Hollywood writer/director in his early sixties. His main residence is in Europe along with his wife and five children. I met Carl as an attendee of a private video lecture I gave on the structure and formation of the multiverse as well as information on its nonhuman inhabitants. He is quite articulate, kindhearted, highly intelligent, and displays an incredible sense of Self-discipline.

Carl is also an intensely private individual who prides himself on exhaustive research for his projects. It is not unusual for him to spend up to five years from start to finish on one of his big-budget movies. The pressure on him to deliver blockbuster films is only exceeded by the expectations he has of himself and his team.

I was hired by Carl to be a consultant on his upcoming film. He is extremely interested in understanding the Greater Reality. He has been incredibly respectful regarding our interactions and with my time. No matter the circumstance, he always maintains an ever-present, genuine curiosity for our work together. I've met his family more than once, and all of them made me feel very welcome.

I received a text from him about a month before he was scheduled to start scouting for locations for his upcoming film. He said he wanted to have a conversation regarding subject matter outside of our current working relationship. We set up a video call for the next morning, and I noted it within my day planner.

The next morning, I got right to business. I made a chai latte with a single shot of espresso and whole milk. I added just a touch of whip cream on the top. Have I mentioned that I enjoy coffee? I flipped open my laptop and logged into my virtual meeting with Carl.

"*Guten Morgen*, heir Carl."

"*Alles klar*, heir RJ."

"It feels like you are in Berlin, my friend."

"Amazing! Yes, I am."

"*Guten Morgen* is pretty much the extent of my Deutsche other than *ich habe zwei Hunde*. It means I have two dogs."

"Very impressive, albeit brief."

"The impressive part is not even remotely true, but you're kind for saying so. What's on your mind?"

"RJ, I don't feel right."

"In what way?"

"I'm off. Way off. I'm not focused like I need to be. Sasha [his wife] and I got to Berlin two days ago. My team is here, essentially, with their significant others. I wanted to take a week before we start running around the world scouting. We shot our first big film right here, way back when."

"You have plenty of time to cut out the noise, drill down, and lock in."

"RJ, I don't even know if I can make this film right now. The script is phenomenal. The cast is as perfect. I love what you added to my understanding, to everybody's understanding, really. But it's like I'm not hungry. It's not life or death for me and that feels weird. Really weird. And dangerous for me."

"That's because you are used to being driven to achieve and succeed in the way that this world has programmed you to. Your identity and Self-worth have been tied to your work. When greater Self-awareness begins to break the addictions and confines of the subconscious, patterned egoic mind, the source of your previous motivation initially wanes."

"That's what I'm concerned about. I can't have that. There is 150 million [dollars] already committed. There's going to be a line of credit for another 100 for print [advertising]. I need to be hyper focused and super motivated."

"Carl, trust yourself. You know what to do and how to do it. Your talents and skills have been honed over dozens of films and nothing can take that away. Your motivation is changing because you are changing."

"I'm getting older by the minute, mate. Yes, I'm changing."

"You don't see things the same way anymore because you don't see yourself in the same way. You have a completely different understanding of earth, the multiverse, what's in it, and our role in the bigger picture. It's a total paradigm shift. It's like somebody pulled the carpet out from under you, and you don't have the same secure footing anymore. It's really given you something to think about, deeply."

"It sure has. How do I get my passion and drive back? It's not just about me. I have investors I have to worry about. I set the tone for the entire project. It's my responsibility to lead the crew and everybody involved. I'm telling you, this time it feels different. I'm seriously concerned."

"How much time do you have, realistically, before you leave to start scouting locations?"

"We have a week here, and I can send my cinematographer, producer, and assistant director with their people ahead for probably another ten days after that. Two and half weeks, realistically."

"That's more than enough time."

"For what, mate? I'm all ears but no clue."

"To find your true motivation by getting to the Self. To do this, you must deprogram your subconscious, patterned, egoic mind. I can show you what to do, but you must do the work. You will never be the same again. Your energy, clarity, focus, and determination will be on a level you have never felt before. If this is what you want, I can show you how to do it."

"RJ, as long as it doesn't entail me dressing up like Little Bo-Peep, I'm in."

I explained to Carl the notebook exercise and the energy diagnostic system. We didn't have the full three weeks, but with Carl's dedication and focus, I was quite confident he would come out the other end with a completely renewed sense of Self and the freed-up energy to go with it. Good thing these teachings do not require any nursery rhyme costumes because clearly this is where Carl has a limitation.

That day, Carl took a flight to Majorca, Spain. He got a hotel right on the water. Per my instruction, he was determined not to have any distractions. He spoke with Sasha before he left and explained to her what he needed to do. She was fully supportive and grabbed a flight back to their California residence.

Working with Carl in this way, within this limited time frame and under extremely stressful circumstances for him personally and professionally, was very challenging, but people have no idea what they are capable of until they are well outside their comfort zone. This situation certainly fit that criterion for Carl on multiple levels.

Seventeen days later, it was the big day. Carl was going to decide whether he could move forward with his project or not. In many ways, there was much more at stake than just a Hollywood blockbuster. Ever since Carl and I met, he had begun to deeply question his views on everything, especially the ones he held regarding himself. This just wasn't about another big movie for Carl, and we both understood that.

I spoke to Carl several times during those past two and a half weeks. His great wealth affords him certain luxuries, and he identified with that lifestyle. The past few months of us working together made him see just how deep his attachments went. He saw how his fame and monetary success affected his family and friends. Now he was seeing just how much it had affected him.

All I want for Carl, for everyone, is liberation and evolution with the greatest efficacy. It was time to see where Carl had landed in this process. Of course, as you well know by now, I would never embark on any journey without imbibing properly. I prepared a hazelnut espresso with salted caramel flakes. And yes, it's divine. I turned on my computer, logged into my virtual meetings, and turned on my computer camera.

"Carl, nice to see you again. Mallorca suits you."

"This place was perfect for the kind of introspection I desperately needed. Great call."

"True excavation was needed, my friend. Tell me where you are at with everything?"

"Mate, I have never felt like this in my entire bloody life. Initially, I was gutted. Now, it's like everything that has been suffocating me has lifted. I've been reborn. I can see better. Everything is crisper, brighter. My heart and mind are clear. Not only am I making this film, but it's also going to be the best film I've ever made."

"I never had a moment's doubt. I am proud of you for being brave enough and determined enough to do what you needed to do."

"Mate, you're bloody spiritual genius. I don't even know what to say, really. Thank you." Tears welled up in his eyes, and his voice trailed off. He was overcome with gratitude. The intensity of it was more than his body could handle.

"You don't have to say anything. Thank you for allowing me to be of service. You allow me to serve my life purpose. Thank you from the bottom of my heart."

We didn't say anything for a long moment. Everything that needed to be shared between us was being said without words. These moments are what stay in my heart for all eternity.

"I do want to hear about the energy diagnostics you did and what you discovered. You already told me about the results from the notebook exercise last week, and those were profound, but I haven't heard about the energy diagnostics."

"I knew I was spending an awful amount of time with my industry friends, my representation, business manager, publicity agents, screenwriters, crew, and it was always about what's next—what other people have lined up. Audience testing, product placement, sponsor-ship opportunities, always trying to get ahead of the curve. Anything and everything so the project is profitable and award worthy. You're defined, you're consumed by what you're working on and what kind of box office and accolades your film can generate."

"By always surrounding yourself with that company and their general area of interest, you cannot help but get caught up in it and consumed by it," I told him.

"Everything was about my fear of becoming irrelevant or losing money, which goes hand in hand. It was totally draining and disem-powering me. I didn't even realize it. I had no idea how negatively impacted I was until I measured it. It was deeply affecting me. I lost my passion."

"Do you know why they call it *Hollywood*, Carl? Because Merlin the Great used to wave his staff made from the holly tree when he would cast his magick spells."

You could see Carl's mind working at light speed, putting together decades of moments and experiences that were now being seen with a completely different perspective. He slowly nodded and a huge smile spread across his face.

"You know what else I realized by doing the energy diagnostics? My life was never about now. Never. I lost my center, and that's why I started to doubt myself. It's why I didn't feel the passion, the drive. Now that I see it, uncovered it, and measured it, I'm never going to spend my energy in the same way again."

"So-called culture, as it pertains to entertainment, is way down-stream of 'what is.' The more you stay true to what is within you, the more tangible that passion and drive to express your authenticity becomes. You're a great storyteller, Carl. Make sure you're clear as to whose and what story you're telling and why."

"I will. There's more I discovered with the energy diagnostics. Like my exhaustive research on everything. I realized how that was providing a terrible return on investment as well. I want to share the whole lot, but I need to arrange transportation to Antarctica. We're thinking about shooting some a bit there."

"That sounds incredibly fascinating, isolating, and absolutely freezing all at the same time."

"Do you want me to join me? I can get you on a private plane here, and we can be on our way to the bone-snapping, frozen tundra in no time."

"Shoot something in the Seychelles or Tahiti, then ask me. Let common sense prevail, my friend."

Carl dedicated himself to these teachings and the results were profound. He is lighter, excited, optimistic, energized, and connected to something deeper within himself than ever before. This kind of transformation and rejuvenation is available and within all of us, always.

He has found deeper meaning and purpose within himself. Not only has his life improved in every way, but it also brought out an even higher quality of artistry within his work. His passion and focus were already legendary, but now it's on an entirely different level.

Carl no longer wastes his attention on anything that doesn't bring the best return on investment. He also deeply understands that the patterned, egoic mind is what confines and hijacks our most precious assets: our sentience and our energy. His ability to transform and bring out the best in himself was achieved through fierce determination, dedication, discipline, and detachment.

Jack

Jack is a makeup artist in his mid-forties and lives in Denver, Colorado. He has two young kids and is recently divorced. Through his rocky marriage, he never allowed himself to pursue his spirituality, nor was he supported in it. He has always had a deep affinity toward mediumship and has always been drawn to non-Western healing modalities.

About six months ago, due to the stress of his divorce and his need to satiate spiritual longings, he reached out to me. He had read my first book, and those new understandings were life changing for him. He was very interested in learning how to unlock his psychic and healing abilities that he has always felt he had.

He booked a private session with me. In his email, he stated that he was very interested in changing careers. He felt stifled and had out-grown his current profession. He wanted to pursue his latent psychic and healing abilities. He also longed for a romantic relationship.

I intuited many epiphanies were on the horizon for Jack. A signif-icant peeling away of the programmed non-Self was needed to tan-gibly see and move through the myriad layers of indentations and identifications. It's work we all must do in order to transcend the various limitations we have imprisoned our unlimited Self within. Jack's true nature and profound abilities are already within him, just like you.

I can also intuit that unless I share what my chosen beverage for the day is, you would be profoundly disappointed! I shall never fail you, my friends. Before my morning session with Jack, I brewed a triple espresso with oat milk, whip, and a dash of caramel syrup. Now we can all proceed properly. I turned on my computer, logged in to Zoom, and joined my scheduled meeting.

"Hi, Jack. Nice to meet you."

"Hi, RJ. I'm trying not to be nervous. It's so weird that I am speak-ing with you."

"Why? There is nothing to be nervous about. This is your hour. I'm happy to go in whatever direction you would like to. I know you read my book and purchased the app. Thank you so much. It really helps our time be more productive when you already have that foun-dation and working knowledge in place."

"Every time I read your book, listen or watch you, everything you are saying, I feel like I already know it. It's so weird."

"That's because the truth is tangible. When you hear truth, it's inner recognition, the deep knowingness. It's already in your heart."

"Yes, that's it! I feel it in my heart. You say everything in such a way that is so easy to grasp."

"Please tell my editor that. It's my pleasure, my love, and my honor to serve. My work is simply a reminder of what is possible for all of us."

"That's what I want to talk to you about. I know so much of what you say is in me. When I was a kid, I used to see and talk to spirits all the time. My mom was super psychic too. I got it from her."

"Your higher intuitive functions have nothing to do with genetics or hereditary traits. They are aspects of what you really are: the Immortal Self. The suit you incarnate into and the family you have chosen to be part of has nothing to do with it."

"Really? I figured it was something that gets passed on, like intelligence, or athleticism, or even cancer, in a weird way."

"You can incarnate into a family that is working on similar things, under similar circumstance, and sometimes at similar levels, but biological family, regarding higher intuitive functionality, is irrelevant. It's just an accepted belief, and like all beliefs, it was born from the conditioned, unawakened mind."

"Wow. I had that totally wrong. I thought it dictated everything."

"Not in terms of what we are talking about. You came into this incarnation with your abilities. We all do. You are your abilities. It's whether you awaken to them or not. It's your human conditioning— your indentations and identifications—that has blanketed any inner recognition of this."

"That makes perfect sense."

"You are still wholly unaware of your incredible healing abilities."

Jack's jaw dropped and his eyes widened. I knew he always felt this inside, but it was time for him to receive confirmation. He needed it as a permission slip to move forward with his life plan.

"Are you serious? I'm a healer?!"

"A profound one. You have always suspected this. Your psychic abilities are part of this skill set."

"You can see this?"

"Yes, but not in the way your physical eyes deceive you. You are longing for a more spiritual existence so you can be in alignment with the Real You. It's why your marriage ended. It's why you seek a change in your profession. It's because those things no longer serve you. They are no longer part of the current section of your life plan. It's why you and I are talking right now."

"Oh my God. This is crazy. You're the one who is supposed to help me with this."

"No, you're the one. God/Source/Creator helps those who help themselves. It will be a matter of your dedication, devotion, and discipline. It always is. You have sought me out as a permission slip for you to be and express what you already are."

Jack's mind was trying to process all this life-changing information. I simply validated what he always felt inside. I can teach him, but I meant it when I said it will be up to him. It's always up to the individual.

"How do we do this, RJ?"

I didn't respond nor did I speak.

"Okay, what do I need to do?"

"Better. The only block is what you put in the way of 'what is.' There is no resistance to anything. You create resistance. It will be a matter of how deep you go in terms of deprogramming your subconscious, patterned, egoic mind and free up your energy. Those comprise the layers of illusion—the indentations and identifications—that you suffer."

"Can you show me what I need to do? I really want my life to be better. I want it to reflect who I really am. I know I have a lot of work to do…but I'm finally ready to do it."

"Are you prepared to question your every action? Are you willing to let go of everything that you hold dear? Are you truly ready to see your ego/mind/identity, warts and all? Don't just say yes, Jack. This is the most important and challenging work you or anyone else can ever do. I do not work with people who aren't all in."

Jack nodded his head slowly as he weighed what I just said. Rarely do I see anyone with the healing abilities Jack has. Abilities he has honed over many lifetimes. I know what it takes to make these aspects of the Self tangibly known and at our command to serve humanity powerfully.

"I am so ready, RJ. This is what I need in my life. I need the Real Me. I'll do whatever it takes to make it happen."

"Now we're on the same page. Let's proceed."

I explained to Jack the notebook exercise and the energy diagnostic system. He was excited and determined to get to work. I reminded him that being open-minded, courageous, truthful, and dedicated were requirements. The moment one of those wanes, growth stops. He reiterated his intention to see it through, and we agreed to speak again in three weeks.

Three weeks later, I was particularly interested to see what Jack discovered. We spend our whole life being programmed. We simultaneously build and believe in the false character we create that goes along with it. It requires perpetual gentle tenacity to deconstruct what we spent our whole life building and believing in.

Jack has truly powerful healing and psychic abilities. Until he sees everything that has prevented those talents from expressing themselves, he and the world will be missing out on something truly needed.

It was time to speak with Jack, so I flipped open my laptop, got out my day planner, and logged in to my first meeting of the day. My delicious, caffeinated beverage for the day was roasted brown rice green tea from Korea with creamer and local honey. I must be channeling my inner barista! Okay, now I was ready to work.

"Hi, Jack. Nice to see you. How have you been?"

"I'm great. It's nice to see you too. I can't wait to share with you what has happened."

"Please do."

"First off, the notebook exercise is the most eye-opening and life-changing thing I have ever done. Ever. My whole life is about my patterned ego mind. I can't believe it. I do nothing truly for myself, my Real Self."

"It's mind-boggling, isn't it? We never realize this, the depth at which we are programmed, because we never dedicate ourselves to this type of Self-inquiry."

"I feel like all the weight and stress of my life has been dematerialized."

"Amazing how much we can change our life in just a few weeks. Great job, Jack. I'm proud of you."

"Thank you so much, RJ. I have never felt this good."

"Tell me about the energy diagnostics you did."

"Yes! I think what I was most surprised by is the return on investment on going out with my friends. It was quite negative. We spent most of our time gossiping, drinking, and talking about past relationships. I never saw how it really affected me."

"Drinking and gossiping are both extremely low frequency. Drinking and drugs, even prescription drugs, erode your auric layers, your larger body of energy, and make you susceptible to psychic attachments and entities."

"Are you serious? I never feel like myself once I start drinking."

"Now you know why. If you could see, from a higher-consciousness perspective, what type of entities hang out at bars, even medical facilities, you would avoid them at all costs. Disincarnate troubled Souls looking to get drunk off your low energies and astral entities looking to feed on you as well. Both can attach themselves to you, and it's deeply unsettling, unhealthy, and dangerous on many levels."

"Is this why I feel so weird and act totally different when I drink?"

"Yes. They call alcohol *spirits* for a reason."

"Wow. I am not drinking anymore."

"A drink or two is fine if you don't have an addiction. Understand your motivation behind heavy or consistent drinking. That is the key. Gossiping creates karma and is best to avoid at all costs."

"I'm going to stop doing that too. I don't like how I feel anyway when I talk about other people. Now that I did the energy diagnostics, I can't deny it. It really led me to something even more impactful."

"What's that?"

"I feel like I spend a lot of time fantasizing and pursuing women. That was a huge negative return on investment. I also saw how much importance and attention I was putting on my looks. Yet another terrible return on investment. All this made me realize I want a deep connection with someone, but if I am so concerned about what I look like, that is exactly the kind of person I will attract."

"So wise, Jack. The subconscious, egoic programming of needing to be in a relationship, to feel complete through validation, was driving your Self-worth. Constant attention on your looks will only attract like-minded people. Now that you know this, you realize why you have not made a deep, spiritual love connection yet. You haven't had your attention dwelling within the Self."

"I finally get it. And now I see it with the energy diagnostics. All the wasted energy going outward. I have totally changed what I put my attention on, and my life has changed already."

"What investments have provided a positive return on investment in regard to your attention?"

"This work! As soon as I started doing this work, my psychic abilities have totally come online. You were right. I can communicate with my deceased little cousin. I even did a reading for a friend so he could talk to his dad who died two years ago from cancer. It's incredible. As soon as I stopped wasting my energy, chasing after my own better looks, a woman, or wanting to drink and gossip and focused my attention on the inner me, all my abilities just exploded."

"You are changing your inner life because you want to grow. It's simple metaphysics. Attention is energy. Put your attention on what you want to flower and grow. You are deprogramming yourself by doing the notebook exercise and freeing up your energy—becoming more powerful—by running the energy diagnostics."

"I had no idea how totally life altering this would be in just three weeks. And that if you do the work, you can see and feel the changes. I'm finally going to be able to change my profession into something that really speaks to me: spiritual work."

"What did you learn about your healing abilities?"

"RJ, I need to talk to you about this. My guides and angels say that you are the one who can help me unlock my healing abilities. They said I can do energy healing like Reiki. Is that true?"

"You're way past Reiki. You can do anything with healing. You have that kind of ability."

"Are you serious?! Can you help me with this?"

"Jack, you are the one who will unlock your healing abilities. I am just a permission slip, remember?"

"Right, yes. I am ready to help myself. Would you assist me in that process?"

"It would be my honor."

Jack is a completely transformed person. He and I spent the next few months working together weekly on my healing course. I instructed him on the higher-consciousness metaphysics of energy healing as I understand and perform them.

Now that Jack has discovered how sacred and precious his attention is, he has learned to focus it on what brings him the greatest return on investment: him being and expressing his True Self. Not coincidentally at all, he is attracting a completely different circle of people. That's because like energies attract like energies. Opposites do not attract.

Jack is doing energy healings and readings for people. He is beginning to support himself in this way. He has put in the work and part of the reward is access to more and more of his True Self. With it are all those natural talents and abilities. Jack needed his True Self in this incarnation, and so does the world.

Vince

Vince is in his early seventies and lives in New York City with his wife of over fifty years. He is a retired accountant with two adult children. He has always been a great athlete and has kept himself in peak physical condition his whole life. A few years ago, he was diagnosed with ALS. His body and mind are declining rapidly. Nothing can be done about it as this is his last exit point for this incarnation.

If anything could be done, I would have done it already. He's also my earthly father.

I certainly didn't have the best relationship with him growing up. He was raised old-school Italian and went to Catholic school through twelfth grade. Our only way of connecting was through sports, namely baseball. Vince was good enough to be a professional baseball player himself, but he was drafted into the army.

He was a standout pitcher prior to being drafted into the military, and he was scouted by the Yankees before leaving for basic training. By the time he got out of the army, my older sister had already been born. A baseball career was not in the cards. He worked during the day and put himself through community college to get an accounting degree.

My father never missed a day of work in thirty-six years. His discipline is legendary. He has been a leader of men in other lifetimes. In this incarnation, he has deeply struggled with emotions and Self-confidence. He text messaged me and asked if we could talk. I sent him a Zoom link so we could video chat. I have always known he would come to me in this life once he stopped seeing me as just his earthly son.

"Dad, how are you doing?"

As soon as he saw me, he became emotional. We made amends many, many years ago. He spent his whole life not being able to deal with his emotions. Only the last few years he has learned to let himself feel them.

"Look at you, RJ. How is it that you are my son..."

He was very emotional. I didn't respond to the statement. I smiled as I scanned his energy field.

"How are you feeling today?"

"I am losing a lot of strength in my arms. But your mom takes care of me."

"That's a challenge. You like to talk with your hands."

We both laughed. Besides having an otherworldly level of Self-discipline, my father has a fantastic deadpan sense of humor.

"What's troubling you, Dad?"

"My sisters and my brother just invited Mom and I to a family get-together."

"And you're stressed about it, yes?"

"I remember when you told me, it must have been twenty-five years ago, how much my family has affected me. Nothing's changed. At least I'm consistent."

"Yes, very. Did you want to speak about this?"

"I want to finally move past it. I've pretty much waited until the end to finally stop being such a coward about it."

"You're not a coward. There's not a single coward on this entire planet. It takes serious courage and guts just to incarnate here. Give yourself some credit."

"Well, since you put it that way. I want to address these things that you teach the world about. I have avoided this my entire life. You are the only person I trust to do this with."

"I'm honored. Just trust yourself and the process."

"RJ, you have no idea how much I love you.

"I do, Dad. I truly do. I love you too."

"There is no way for me to express how proud I am of you. You are everything I wish to be …"

Frankly, this was too much for me. My heart was breaking. My dad could never really see me at all until recently. I was always too much for him. I knew he didn't have much longer left in this incarnation. And I knew how much guilt he harbored, how much love he kept hidden from himself and from me.

"I can show you what to do. Are you sure you want to do this? You are going to learn things about yourself that have been hidden deep within the recesses of your mind and body of energy your entire life."

"I do. I need to do this. I'm determined to do it."

"Are you able to hold a pen and write?"

"I have voice to text on my phone. I use that."

"Then let's begin."

I explained to my dad the notebook exercise and the energy diagnostic system. He was absolutely fascinated with the entire process and how it reveals the patterned, subconscious, egoic mind. My dad has heard me talk about these things for a very long time. Other than the magick tricks to instantly meditate, this was really the first time he was going to dedicate himself to any of my teachings.

I was excited for him to make these incredible discoveries about himself. This moment was inevitable, and even though his lifetime was nearing its completion, some of his most important work was just about to begin.

I text messaged him support over the next few weeks. I knew that was all he needed. Once he makes up his mind to do something, he does it. If he gives his word, you can bet your life he will follow through. It's an incredibly admirable quality to have. My father also stopped cursing about twenty years ago. I have never, in my entire life, heard him say anything negative about anyone except about himself.

It was time for our session together. I was proud of him for doing this work. I knew it was needed before he leaves this incarnation. I am so grateful I am allowed to teach these things and be here for him, and for all of you. I didn't bother with a drink when the day came. I flipped opened my laptop and logged into my virtual meeting with my dad.

"How are you doing?"

"I never thought this was possible. My body is shutting down, but I feel free."

"I know exactly what you mean. I'm so happy to hear that. Tell me about what the last three weeks were like."

"There are no words to describe how different I feel about everything. In the beginning, when I was doing the notebook exercise, I could not believe how everything I think, feel, and do was based upon my programming, my ego. It's not possible to put this experience into words until you have experienced it firsthand."

"Exactly. Mental understandings are not the truth about anything. We can learn from reading, but we only know through love."

"It's like my thinking mind has disappeared. I feel such joy and love. I never thought this was ever possible for me. I can't believe I waited seventy-five years to get a clue."

"When doesn't matter except to the ego mind. It's only ever now. How do you feel physically?"

"I feel like I got lighter, and my body isn't even me. I know what you mean now. It's like a suit. Just like I what I wore every day to go to work."

"Precisely. What did you learn about yourself? How do you feel about yourself now?"

"Like I have never known myself. I never allowed myself to get to know the Real Me. Now I realize I never accepted myself. The pressures of my identity overwhelmed me emotionally. It's why I only had two forms of expression: rage and silence. I never accepted the Real Me, and it's why I never could see or accept the Real You."

It's like our entire lifetime together was being healed. I didn't speak because this was exactly what he needed. Right then, in this silence between us, was the most profound exchange of love we had ever shared in this lifetime. I didn't want the moment to ever end. Truth be told, I couldn't really speak.

"I did the energy diagnostics too. Once I started to realize the beauty of this teaching, I stopped paying attention to anything other than what I feel in my heart for Louise [my mom], you, and Christine [my sister]. I haven't done anything since but feel that. Thank you, Son."

I had been trying to stay detached, but I couldn't anymore. I began to weep. My dream had come true. My father had liberated himself from his suffering. The feelings were so intense, they overwhelmed me.

There are no words to describe what this moment meant to my father and me.

He left his body two months later. He is with me as I write this. He knows how much I love him. I told him he is welcome here anytime. My door is always open.

Summary

The energy diagnostic system gives you a robust and repeatable process for total awareness regarding how you are spending your energy. Because you now have awareness like never before, this gives you the ability to make powerful adjustments without having to repeatedly experience poor results. If you are not experiencing or manifesting what it is that you are trying to achieve, you now have the tools to deeply understand yourself better, pivot when needed, and create powerfully.

In addition to expanded inner awareness, greater flexibility in life force allotment, and empowerment as it relates to the reality you wish to create, you also have a quantifiable metric on your energetic return on investment. You never again have to wonder which people, situations, or activities aren't healthy for you and which ones truly are. The energy diagnostic system takes out all the guesswork. Now you can focus on creating the life you truly desire instead of leaking your energy on doubting, ruminating, or projecting.

Use the energy diagnostic system like your new metaphysical to-do list. The more acutely aware you are of how you spend your energy and its subsequent return on investment, the more successful your life will be, period. You will be able to initiate dramatic and emphatic shifts in your life that would normally take years, decades, or perhaps never happen at all.

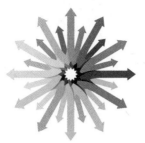

Conclusion

To own your own mind is the greatest gift and the most beautiful treasure. No one can give that to you or do it for you. I have, through this book, paved the way for you to do just that. The notebook exercise, energy diagnostic system, and activities to integrate the Real You are yours forever. Nothing can ever take away what always remains: the Real You.

Recognizing what is not authentically you is the first step. Having the expertise and tools to do just that is real power. You have now seen and let go of all that holds you back. You have now discovered how to supremely focus your energy for the greatest return on investment regarding having a successful, fulfilling, and happy life. Learning the simple activities that effortlessly integrate the Real You back into your human life is the elixir for all that ails your Soul.

What you have discovered and experienced by deprogramming your subconscious mind cannot be replaced by beliefs, concepts, ideologies, or bodily sensations. That is because what you have discovered is the Real You. You no longer need beliefs, concepts, ideologies, or bodily sensations to give you what you already have before any of those things were ever created. Your freedom.

Use this book to liberate yourself and experience a superior quality of life. The dedication, courage, honesty, and discipline required to meet the Real You is a microcosm of your entire evolutionary cycle. Once the work is done, it's time to come home. I am waiting for you there.

You have all my love and attention, now and forever.

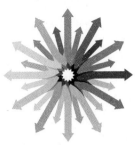

Glossary

awareness: Pure, unsullied perception itself sans analysis; the eyes of the Immortal Self. Embedded within pure awareness, action takes place. It is the Self's depth of unconditional love and timeless wisdom, which is sentience. Attention automatically activates the divine intelligence, or sentience, within the fabric of awareness itself.

being: Any individualized unit of consciousness, Self-awareness, or sentience that was created organically through the natural attraction of like charged energies drawn together, which forms a larger, more capable, and robust individual unit. Not the same as an entity, which is a manipulated creation by a higher intelligence.

consciousness: The rudimentary intelligent life force that animates energy. Consciousness is expressed in infinite degrees and amounts. Consciousness has the potentiality of evolving and becoming Self-aware through the accumulation and commingling of other similarly charged energies. This leads to consciousness potentially becoming Self-aware, which can, in turn, lead to the development of sentient Self-awareness. Sentience accrues via experiences through the use of imagination.

ego/mind/identity (EMI): The ego/mind/identity (EMI) has been commonly referred to as the ego, or ego mind, or false identity.

The belief-based egoic mind is the individual's Self-created totality of misperceptions, misunderstandings, and misidentifications. This includes the Self's misidentification with the perceiver and experiencer of sensory perceptions, the physical body, which binds its awareness within the confining delusion of limiting body consciousness. Every sensory perception is then seen and subsequently decoded only in relation to the false Self-program running. The egoic mind is a limitation program, since all sensory perceptions are limited, and therefore so is the logic-based and linear-bound intellect. It is a product of a low-frequency environment, and its primary resultant side effect produces a stupor-like state we call thinking. It is a limitation program that runs by thinking.

emotion: Energy in motion based upon identification with phenomena such as thoughts, images, and experiences. The more we see the false self in it, the more we bathe the experience in emotion. This occurs in a near-instantaneous arrangement (because of the deep programming of the ego/mind/identity) of core hierarchical beliefs regarding the foundational elements of its personal relationship with the thought or image. The more emotional the reaction, the greater the sense of identification to the false self as it relates to the image, thought, memory, or experience.

energy: Life substance that carries the potentiality of infinite possibility.

entity: Any individualized unit of consciousness, sentience, or sentient Self-awareness that was intentionally created by others. Technically the Total Self is an entity created by its Totality, or Higher Self. Humans are entities created by their Total Self. The Total Self is an entity created by its Totality, or Higher Self. Our Totality, or Higher Self, is a creation of our Source, or Creator, which makes it an entity as well. Our Source, or Creator, was created by the Absolute, or the All There Is, which makes our Source and other Sources entities as well.

free will: The "experience" of freedom as it pertains to perceivable choices in order to evolve oneself; the human experiment is the experiment in individualized free will as an avenue for the most expedient route for the evolution of individual and collective consciousness, or, more specifically, for the accrual of sentience; at the deepest levels, it is an illusion, as once creation is set into motion, absolute free will is no longer possible.

frequency: An assignation of energy; a specific rate or environment that energy exists within and vibrates in accordance with.

gnosis: Knowledge of Self or Self-knowledge. The only true knowledge that exists.

higher intuitive functions: The expressions, attributes, abilities, or "talents" of the Self, such as clairsentience, claircognizance, clairvoyance, telepathy, etc.

indentation: Any non-germane force or encroachment of energy within our body of energies that has become stuck, embedded, or patterned within our naturally unsullied energies.

identification (misidentification): The cause of all suffering; the misunderstanding that occurs when infinite Creator Awareness, such as the Self, misidentifies itself with anything that can be perceived, such as beliefs, thoughts, emotions, experiences, memories, or what has been learned. This includes the "perceiver" and "experiencer" of sensory perceptions, the genetic entity, as well as the meanderings of the intellect.

incarnate: The temporary experience that a collective life force, Self-aware being, or conscious entity has within the lower frequencies of the physical universe.

intention: The harnessing of energy, or qi; a fixed focal point of energy within the creative process.

judgment: The opposite of unconditional love; nonacceptance; the belief-based ego/mind/identity; the egoic false Self-imposing its sense of self upon the divine Self, others, and all sensory-perceived stimuli.

knowing: The tangible recognition of inner alignment or truth, not mental machinations or emotional roilings.

magick: The ability to harness and manipulate higher frequential energies that exist beyond physical sensory perceptions by utilizing pure desire and unbroken intention. This can be augmented by the use of higher intuitive functions.

meditation: The space between thoughts; the cessation of the egoic mind running its program of limitations we call thinking. When done properly, meditation annihilates the misperception that we are merely human or limited in any way. The freeing of awareness from ordinary sensory perceptions, the limiting intellect, and debilitating body consciousness.

metaphysics: Hidden from the five senses and therefore the processing of the logical and linear intellect are the inner workings, depth, function, and interplay of sentience and energy; a more holistic and accurate understanding of existence itself.

multi-frequential: Energy and/or sentience that simultaneously exists within multiple frequencies concurrently and in parallel.

reality: The Self-directed relationship an individual creates in regard to all sensory stimuli; individualized, group, or collective experience seen from a similar state of understanding.

(the) Real You: The Self.

Reiki: An ancient healing modality originally created by an Ascended Master in which the practitioner, through the harnessing of their intention, uses their energetic and physical body as a conduit of higher-frequency energy for healing aided by the utilization of specific symbols.

Self: Sentience; the amount, level, or weight of our love and wisdom.

Self-inquiry: The direct introspection into the nature of the Self.

Self-mastery: The Self, while projected from its Totality, existing in a state of knowing itself at the very depths and origination of its existence during its incarnation; the ability to transcend the Self-imposed limitations of the egoic mind, body consciousness, and localized frequential environment as well as the ability to command energies within and outside the Total Self at will. This exalted state is always in direct proportion and relation to the level or amount of sentience that is the Self. Authentic Self-mastery is an extraordinarily rare occurrence and is the domain of very specific incarnations of Masters.

sentience: What we really are; the Self; the amount, level, or weight of timeless wisdom and unconditional love expressed as an individualized unit or collective; divine, loving intelligence not bound by space or time.

Source: Our Creator, or God. We exist within Source's creation called the multiverse, which is within Source itself. Everything within our entire multiverse is a creation, whether direct or indirect, of our Source with the tiniest of exceptions we call the Ascended Masters.

thought: The movement of the past; the movement of memory, experience, and so-called knowledge. All thought is the past, including the so-called future, as the past must be recalled to conceptualize a future. Thinking is faltering itself and is simply a byproduct of experiencing a low-frequency environment—the opposite of knowing.

Totality: Sentience—what we really are—given a complement or body of energy to create with; our individualized sentience and its complement of energy projected from our Totality. What we totally are even while incarnate—not the person within the human experience but what originally gives birth to any temporary experiences of personhood, including personhood itself. Commonly referred to as the Soul.

transcendence: The moving into a more holistic state of awareness; a rise in frequential being-ness beyond a limited understanding of that which is currently experienced.

transmutation: The enhancement, or augmentation, from that which is into that which can be; the foundation of alchemy.

wisdom: The direct, experiential knowingness that occurs only though observation; the divine intelligence of the Self; the timeless knowingness that is part of the very fabric of the Immortal Self; the eternally applicable level of gnosis woven within the fabric of awareness itself.

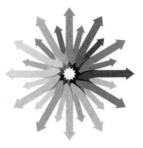

Appendix
Summary of Book

In part 1 of *Change Your Mind*, you learned how to deprogram the patterned, subconscious, egoic mind by using the revolutionary notebook exercise and, in doing so, finally met the Real You!

This extraordinarily powerful yet incredibly simple Self-inquiry journal exercise brings your subconscious programming into view of your conscious mind. This engenders permanent change and recognition of the Real You!

Quick Summary of the Notebook Exercise

In doing the notebook exercise, I wrote everything down that I was doing. Every notion, action, and behavior. I needed to write it all down so I could see it myself. I wrote down everything I was experiencing or compelled to do. I would then relentlessly question and demand to know the core motivation driving the behavior. I needed to consciously know and tangibly understand my motivation behind every notion. Until I could tangibly see why RJ was the way he was, I would never be able to fully understand nor transcend him. I demanded my own liberation and decided I would stop at nothing to experience my total freedom and Self-realization. Here is the very first example from one of the notebooks I have kept all these years:

Quick Example of the Notebook Exercise

> *Question:* Why I am brushing my hair?
>
> *Answer:* So it looks good.
>
> *Question:* Why do I care if my hair looks good?
>
> *Answer:* So other people find me attractive.
>
> *Question:* Why do I care if other people find me attractive?
>
> *Answer:* Because I get a sense of my own Self-worth based upon other people's opinion of me.

These types of revelations will completely change your mind and your life by simply questioning the seemingly mundane thoughts/emotions/actions/behaviors you do habitually.

12 Limiting Habits

Next, we learned the top twelve limiting habits of the subconscious mind. They are as follows:

#1: Thinking

#2: Identifying

#3: Reacting

#4: Needing to Be Productive

#5: Seeking Security

#6: Craving Stimulation

#7: Judgment

#8: Chasing Pleasure

#9: Seeking Approval/Validation

#10: Asking for Permission

#11: Needing Attention

#12: Needing to Be Right

By seeing these things for what they are—not born of the Real You—it allows you to finally understand your low-frequency programmed habits and finally move past them.

25 Signs of Dissolving Your Egoic Mind

Next, you discovered the top twenty-five signs you are dissolving your subconscious, patterned, egoic mind. Here they are again:

- You desire alone time.
- You feel like you have less in common with people.
- Your hobbies and interests change.
- You cherish simple pleasures more than before.
- You are less negative and not as adversely affected by the world.
- You no longer see anyone or anything in the same way as before.
- You no longer believe in what you are told to believe.
- You feel the desire to help wake up others.
- You lose interest in partying, group gatherings, and gossip.
- Your circle of friends gets smaller.
- You no longer label yourself through identifications.
- You are more intuitive.
- You become calmer and more introspective.
- Everything you thought you knew or believed in no longer seems true.
- Career interests may change.
- Your connection and affinity for nature increases.
- Intimate personal relationships may end, evolve, or transform.
- You seek inner truth rather than beliefs and opinions.
- You desire better mental and emotional health.
- You are more protective of your energy.
- You value yourself and others far more.
- You don't crave constant stimulation and distractions.
- You are less scared by so-called failure.

- You are more determined and less deterred.
- Your highest desire is to be at peace and to feel happy.

Becoming the Real You

In part 2, you learned how to express the Real You by becoming aware of its thirteen universal qualities. They are as follows:

#1: Patience

#2: Talents and Abilities

#3: Determination

#4: Joy

#5: Acceptance

#6: Wisdom

#7: Contentment

#8: Creativity

#9: Spontaneity

#10: Purpose

#11: Forgiveness

#12: Love

#13: Gratitude

Here is a two-week activity that promotes the tangible experience of the universal qualities of the Real You.

Day #1: Patience

Have a conversation with someone without interrupting them or thinking about formulating a response while they are speaking. Take time to perform an activity that promotes patience, such as fishing, gardening, writing, or assembling a puzzle.

Day #2: Talents and Abilities

Make time today to create something that is near and dear to your heart and give it away. It can be anything: a meal, a drawing, a handwritten letter, etc.

Day #3: Determination

Make a promise to yourself when you wake up and do it that very day. It could be to clean the garage, to meditate, to go for a walk, to take a drive, or to call a loved one. Set the intention and follow through.

Day #4: Joy

You are joy. Sometimes you need to break your habitual patterns in order to give yourself the permission slip needed to bring it out! Laugh and play with your grandchildren, relatives, siblings, parents, coworkers, companion entities, friends, etc.

Day #5: Acceptance

Let the mind become so still that the ebb and flow of all life is directly and tangibly experienced. No analysis, no expectation, no rumination. Meditate, do yoga, stretch, lose yourself in pure observation, and breathe deeply from the diaphragm.

Day #6: Wisdom

Self-reflect by journaling on how you spent your energy today (thoughts, emotions, actions, and behaviors). Did you spend your day thinking/doing, and about what? Self-reflect on how you were being while interacting with people. Were you kind, pushy, loving, short-tempered, determined, attentive, etc.?

Day #7: Contentment

Turn off your egoic mind and lose yourself in the play of nature. Sit under a tree and watch waves crash onto the shore or observe dogs playing, birds flying, squirrels gathering nuts, or fish swimming.

Day #8: Creativity

Make something—anything. It doesn't matter as long as it's reflective of the Real You. Draw, paint, cook or bake, write a song or poem, plant a flower, write an email, dance, create an online course, write a fantasy short story, make a collage, etc.

Day #9: Spontaneity

Without planning, whatever you are most excited about doing in the moment, simply do it. This is one way to remember what it's like to be free of the programmed mind. Go to that movie you have wanted to see, the museum, or the farmers' market. Go see your friend or relative, take a balloon ride, ride go karts, attend a sports game, go on a day trip, start your miniature garden, etc.

Day #10: Purpose

Ask yourself, "What is the single most important driving force in my life?" Once you have your answer, do something today that you have never done in service to that. Use your imagination. Don't think outside the box—remove the box—and make it happen!

Day #11: Forgiveness

Beginning today and moving forward, look in the mirror and say to yourself, "I forgive you." Mean it when you say it. Say it ten times, sincerely, and watch what happens.

Day #12: Love

Give something away, whether it is your time, a gift, energy, money, food, a family heirloom, know-how, and neither expect nor accept anything in return. Make the gift something that comes directly from your heart that you know someone needs and would appreciate. Take yourself out of the equation. Stay attuned to this feeling all day and all night.

Day #13: Gratitude

Make "Thank You" your mantra. Connect with the words and say them again and again. Watch what happens. Pure magick!

48-Hour Retreat Tips to Meet the Real You!

One fun and effective way to deprogram the subconscious mind is to remove yourself from your familiar surroundings. Familiarity breeds comfort and the subconscious, patterned, egoic mind is built upon what it is familiar with—even if what's familiar is very uncomfortable, upsetting, or stressful.

Although not necessary, going camping by the local river, getting a hotel room or even an Airbnb for the weekend is a fantastic way to set yourself up for success while doing your forty-eight-hour weekend challenge if you can leave home.

While you will still follow the guidelines of chapter 3's notebook challenge during your forty-eight-hour retreat, here are the top four ways to accelerate, condense, and supercharge your subconscious deprogramming to meet the Real You!

Turn Off Your Phone!

Turning off your phone/computer removes the primary distractions (technology) that keep you from truly getting to know the Real You. In a section of your notebook, keep track of all the times you unconsciously reach for your phone to scroll, research, shop, post, message someone, or take a photo. Write it down and question why you are really doing it.

No Television

Most of us use TV/movie watching to numb, procrastinate, distract, or entertain ourselves rather than get to know our own completeness, resourcefulness, creativity, and ever-present inner peace and love. Instead of TV watching, practice meditation and notebook the thoughts/emotions that arise from within the subconscious, patterned, egoic mind. You can even inquire if some of those identifications/beliefs were things that you simply bought into because you saw them on television/online.

Get a Mirror

This is not for you to obsess over your hair, worry about a wrinkle, or panic because of a blemish. Instead, each day I want you to stand in front of a mirror (or hold one in your hand), look yourself in the eyes, and say "I love you." Say it ten times. You must look into your eyes, connect with yourself, and mean it when you say, "I love you." Whatever thoughts or emotions arise from this, notebook them and drill down on them like an archaeologist digging for a lost buried treasure (the Real You!)

Go On a Nature Walk

Moving your body while connecting with nature is an elixir for grounding, rejuvenation, and purification. Take in the beauty and wonder of your natural surroundings. As your state of being and thought patterns begin to change, stop and notebook what comes to you. Exercising and notebooking in nature gives you the permission to stop focusing on what's at the forefront of your patterned, subconscious, egoic mind. This gives you a wonderful opportunity to deprogram. Take advantage of it while reconnecting with your own true nature.

How to Run Your Energy Diagnostic System

In part 3, you learned the fun energy diagnostics to balance our energy bank account to maintain the Real You! You also learned how to manage and balance your energy regarding personal relationships, activities, and events so you can always be mindful of how you are operating.

You will ask yourself a series of five simple yet illuminating questions prior to engaging, during, and post engagement and record your answers.

At the end of each series of five questions, you will tally your points. The result will be a tangible and objective answer as to whether it cost you energy (disempowered) and dropped your frequency or revitalized (empowered) and/or raised your frequency.

With your new simple yet incredibly effective energy diagnostic system, you will know if the return on investment of your most precious asset—energy in the form of your attention—was worth the expenditure.

You are going to use your energy diagnostic system for three separate categories: activities, people, and circumstances/events.

There are four ways a human being can express itself: emotionally, mentally, verbally, and physically. We are going to be using these fundamental forms of expressions to measure our state of being before, during, and after our engagement.

In order to assess your purely energetic state of being, we will be using our inner voice (the pure life force given breath through speech) to capture that data. Get ready because what you are about to discover on how you spend your most precious resource will change your mind and your entire life.

You can either create a note on your phone or a computer, use the notebook from the previous exercises, or use a brand-new energy diagnostics notebook. Whatever you pick, divide it into three separate categories: activities, people, and events/circumstances.

Here's What It Looks Like

Before engaging, write down:

- How do I feel emotionally leading up to …?
- What is my thought process leading up to …?
- How do I feel energetically (inner voice) leading up to …?
- How do I feel physically leading up to …?

During engagement, write down:

- How do I feel emotionally during …?
- What is my thought process during …?
- How do I feel energetically (inner voice) while engaged in/ with …?
- How do I feel physically while engaged in/with …?

Post engagement, write down:

- How do I feel emotionally after …?
- What is my thought process after …?

- How do I feel energetically (inner voice) after…?
- How do I feel physically after…?

These written answers will give you great insight into your state of being. They will also clarify your entire experience in an entirely new way. You will no longer walk away after some form of engagement not fully aware and mindful of what you brought to the table, how you engaged, and what your takeaway was.

How to Balance Your Energy Bank Account

You are now ready to calculate your energetic scoring. The ultimate purpose is to discover how to always maintain a positive flow into your energy bank account. Recognizing and quantifying what empowers or disempowers you is essential in the quality of life you experience as well as your new unleashed ability to create it. Attention/energy is your most precious and sacred resource. You are about to learn how to spend it wisely with a proper return on investment.

Low-Frequency Checklist/Scoring

Yes	No	Question
		Do I feel drained/tired/depleted?
		Do I feel down or depressed?
		Am I left feeling frustrated, angry, or a little hostile?
		Do I find myself immediately reaching for something to make me feel better?
		Do I feel like I need to tell someone to get guidance/feel better/validation?

Yes = 1 point
No = 0 points

Give yourself a score:
0 points: Engaging in this does not have a low-frequency effect on me.

1–2 points: Engaging in this is somewhat low frequency.

3 points: This is having a low-frequency effect on me.

4–5 points: This is having an extremely low-frequency effect and
is unhealthy for me on various levels.

High-Frequency Checklist/Scoring

Yes	No	Question
		Do I feel energized and inspired?
		Do I feel happy?
		Do I feel centered and content?
		Do I feel more empowered?
		Do I feel more positive and determined?

Yes = 1 point

No = 0 points

Give yourself a score:

0 points: Engaging in this does not have a high-frequency effect
on me.

1–2 points: Engaging in this is somewhat high frequency.

3 points: This is having a significant high-frequency effect on me.

4–5 points: This is having an extremely high-frequency effect
and is healthy for me on various levels.

Look at your written answers and compare the two scores. You
will know definitively and quantifiably what gives you the greatest
return on investment of your attention and what you need to remove
from your life.

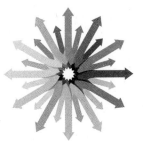

Bibliography

Associated Press. "Americans Are the Unhappiest They've Been in 50 Years, Poll Finds." NBC News. June 16, 2020. https://www .nbcnews.com/politics/politics-news/americans-are-unhappiest -they-ve-been-50-years-poll-finds-n1231153.

Bethune, Sophie. "APA: U.S. Adults Report Highest Stress Level Since Early Days of the COVID-19 Pandemic." American Psychological Association. February 2, 2021. https://www.apa.org/news /press/releases/2021/02/adults-stress-pandemic.

Drah, Hermina. "29 Disturbing Stress Statistics & Facts to Check Out in 2022." *Disturb Me Not* (blog). January 14, 2022. https:// disturbmenot.co/stress-statistics/.

"How Your Subconscious Mind Creates Reality," Inevitable You. Accessed February 24, 2023. http://inevitableyou.com /how-your-subconscious-mind-creates-reality/.

To Write to the Author

If you wish to contact the author or would like more information about this book, please write to the author in care of Llewellyn Worldwide Ltd. and we will forward your request. Both the author and the publisher appreciate hearing from you and learning of your enjoyment of this book and how it has helped you. Llewellyn Worldwide Ltd. cannot guarantee that every letter written to the author can be answered, but all will be forwarded. Please write to:

RJ Spina
℅ Llewellyn Worldwide
2143 Wooddale Drive
Woodbury, MN 55125-2989

Please enclose a Self-addressed stamped envelope for reply,
or $1.00 to cover costs. If outside the U.S.A., enclose
an international postal reply coupon.

Many of Llewellyn's authors have websites with additional information and resources. For more information, please visit our website at http://www.llewellyn.com.

Notes

Notes

Notes